"My recollections of Dr. Barry Gordon hark back to his days in hematology, before he decided that his first love, general internal medicine, was his destiny. He is an Avant Garde thinker."

"My discussions with Dr. Gordon about the possible role testosterone deficiency may play in pulmonary problems in the aged have been very interesting. Hopefully his book will lead to a serious evaluation of the hormone and its effects."

—Martin Bernstein, M.D.

Dr. Bernstein is the former Chief of Pulmonary Disease at Maimonides Medical Center and Beth Israel Hospital, Kings Highway Division, and a Clinical Assistant Professor of Medicine at SUNY Downstate Medical Center College of Medicine.

"Dr. Barry Gordon makes interesting and thought provoking observations about the treatment of heart failure with testosterone. His nicely written clinical vignettes, culled from his extensive experience, give insight into the impact of illness on the patient. In this age of clinical guidelines and 'cookbook medicine', it is refreshing to hear independent ideas towards the goal of improving health."

—Howard Newhouse, M.D.

Dr. Newhouse is a Board Certified Attending Cardiologist at Beth Israel Hospital, and a Fellow of the American College of Cardiology.

Dr. Gordon's thoughts are always interesting and provocative. I feel this publication will stimulate investigation into his more controversial theories.

—H. Barry Opell, M.D.

Dr. Opell is the Chief of Urology at New York Community Hospital of Brooklyn.

"The therapeutic use of testosterone derivatives to enhance strength and sexuality in people with gross deficiency syndromes is well established. To use these substances to improve performance in humans without obvious abnormalities is a novel approach which seems to have merit in selected individuals. Dr. Gordon's approach deserves further consideration and may be an answer to many psycho/skeletal/sexual problems. The downsides of sex hormone therapy must also be evaluated."

—Gabriel Spergel, M.D.

Dr. Spergel is the Chief of Endocrinology at New York Community Hospital and an Associate Clinical Professor of Medicine at Weill Cornell Medical College.

The Idea that muscle and metabolic function may be favorably affected by an increase in levels of testosterone is an intriguing and plausible concept that could be subjected to controlled study.

—N. Lawrence Wayne, M.D.

Dr. Wayne is an endocrinologist, the former Director of the Department of Long Term Care Medicine at Kingsbrook Jewish Medical Center, and Assistant Professor of Medicine at SUNY Downstate Medical Center College of Medicine.

Testosterone Deficiency:
The Hidden Disease

Testosterone Deficiency: The Hidden Disease

✦

A major Health Issue for Every Woman—Every Man

E. Barry Gordon MD
Author of "Get Well, Stay Well"

iUniverse, Inc.
New York Lincoln Shanghai

Testosterone Deficiency: The Hidden Disease
A major Health Issue for Every Woman—Every Man

iUniverse books may be ordered through booksellers or by contacting:

iUniverse
2021 Pine Lake Road, Suite 100
Lincoln, NE 68512
www.iuniverse.com
1-800-Authors (1-800-288-4677)

The information, ideas, and suggestions in this book are not intended as a substitute for professional medical advice. Before following any suggestions contained in this book, you should consult your personal physician. Neither the author nor the publisher shall be liable or responsible for any loss or damage allegedly arising as a consequence of your use or application of any information or suggestions in this book.

ISBN-13: 978-0-595-41494-9 (pbk)
ISBN-13: 978-0-595-67914-0 (cloth)
ISBN-13: 978-0-595-85844-6 (ebk)
ISBN-10: 0-595-41494-X (pbk)
ISBN-10: 0-595-67914-5 (cloth)
ISBN-10: 0-595-85844-9 (ebk)

Printed in the United States of America

Dedicated to my wife, Alicia, without whose love, understanding, great patience, and many contributions, this book would not have been possible.

Contents

Acknowledgements

I take this opportunity to express my gratitude to, first and foremost, my patients. They not only had enough faith in my judgment to ignore the prevailing common opinions on the subject of testosterone, and act on my advice, but also willingly spent the time and effort to dredge out and relate the last nuances of what they were feeling and experiencing.

I also want to thank my colleagues whose kind comments are quoted here.

There were many times when I feared that my observations were so astonishing, and my conclusions so unorthodox, that they might be the product of borderline dementia. While these learned gentlemen maintained a healthy professional questioning of my ideas, and still do, the interest they showed in my reasoning always quickly restored my self-confidence.

I especially want to thank Mr. Philip Garippa for his enthusiastic appreciation of each new finding, for his support for my evolving conjectures, and for his confidence in the legitimacy of my efforts to uncover the consequences of testosterone deficiency.

Preface

A few years ago I began working on a second edition of my book, 'Get Well, Stay Well', published in 1988. I had learned some very interesting things about testosterone during the preceding five or six years and that hormone was supposed to have been nothing more than an additional chapter in the book. As the writing was progressing, however, I was also treating more and more patients in my medical practice with testosterone. It seemed there was no end to the remarkable and unexpected things I was uncovering about the adverse health effects of testosterone deficiency, and to the numbers of my patients who had symptoms of this deficiency. The subject ultimately reached a point of such breadth and importance that I decided that a book exclusively about testosterone deficiency health issues was warranted.

My purpose in writing this book, therefore, is to share my experiences, conclusions, beliefs, and speculations, about the role testosterone plays in the overall well-being of adult males and females, young and old. This includes both sexual health and, even more importantly, as I've discovered, non-sexual health. I must emphasize that I present observation, opinion, and my own case reports. Nothing in this book is the product of controlled medical studies. I do, however, profoundly hope that this book results in many such studies being stimulated and undertaken.

1

What is Testosterone?

Testosterone therapy has been getting a lot of publicity lately, and rightly so. The hormone has a substantial effect on many facets of the human body and mind. Most of the media hype has been about either its considerable energizing sexual effects, or its negative, illegal, overuse to promote bodybuilding and enhance athletic performance. I have the sense that because of these two areas of notoriety the hormone itself has taken on something of a sordid, sleazy, aura. This is very unfortunate. While sexual health is certainly very important to our physical and mental well-being, not to mention our personal relationships, during the past years I've come to recognize and understand that the health consequences of having a deficiency in this hormone are very common, and can be far more serious than simply losing sexual desire, ability, and enjoyment. Hypogonadism (hypo-gonad-ism = testosterone deficiency) is an extremely common condition that is very often the cause of, or a great contributor to, disease, debility, and even, ultimately, death. It would be regrettable for anyone to deny themselves the multiple beneficial effects of replacing a deficiency in this hormone because of its titillating name or popular illegal use.

Testosterone is a "steroid" hormone, and the best way to begin a discussion about that hormone is to first impart an understanding of the word, "steroid". This descriptive chemical term has become very well known and well recognized during recent decades. People use it frequently, but almost no non-professional understands what the word means. My patients always have something of a look of confusion and uncertainty on their faces when they use the word, as in, "That's a steroid, isn't it?" I reply, "Yes it is. What's a steroid?" They shrug because they really have no idea.

To put it simply, in the hormonal sense "steroid" defines a class of hormones that are derived from the parent compound cholesterol. There are many different steroid hormones, and the different steroid hormones have markedly different, often even opposite effects. So when you encounter people expressing an opinion about "steroids" as if they were a single entity, you'll know that they have absolutely no idea what they're talking about.

The steroid hormones are made in the ovaries, the testes, and the adrenal glands (hormone glands on top of the kidneys). The main steroid hormones made by the adrenal glands are necessary for life, and that gland continues to secrete them during our entire lifespan. The steroid hormone, cortisol (a form of cortisone), for example, is vital. If our adrenal glands stopped secreting cortisol we would die. This disease is called Addison's Disease. In significant excess, however, cortisone is catabolic (biologically destructive). It has the potential to have a marked deteriorating effect on the body. It can promote or cause diabetes, severely depress the immune system, thin bones (osteoporosis), and markedly weaken muscles. It erodes the general structure of the body.

This minimal discussion of cortisone would not be complete unless the reader is left with an accurate appreciation of its side effects. Please note that I used the term, "significant excess". The destructive side effects of cortisone treatments are both time and dose related. Many people shrink in horror from the thought of getting a "cortisone shot". Others have the impression that there are only so many cortisone shots you can get during the course of a year, or even a lifetime. The reality is that the amount of cortisone that actually gets into the blood from one or two shots is trivial, and the effects of most forms of cortisone injections are completely gone in a month.

The main steroid hormones made by the ovaries and testes are testosterone, estrogen, and progesterone, the reproductive hormones. Unlike cortisol these hormones are not necessary for us to remain alive, and unlike the adrenal glands, the ovaries and testes do not secrete their hormones during our entire lifespan. If they did this book wouldn't have been written.

The above are some of the naturally occurring steroid hormones. There also exist many synthetic steroid hormones. These have been chemically altered to enhance or decrease some characteristic of the parent hormone. Prednisone, methylprednisolone, and dexamethisone, for example, are all cortisone type hormonal drugs. They all have almost the same basic characteristics of the naturally occurring cortisol, but are much more powerful and are used in a variety of diseases. One example of a medical use for a synthetic testosterone derivative is the hormone nandrolone which has been on the market for decades. It possesses the bone marrow stimulating qualities of testosterone which increase production of red blood cells in certain cases of anemia as is discussed in a later chapter, but doesn't have the sexual or hair growth stimulating effects.

When it comes to testosterone, it might well be that most of its synthetic derivatives have been made by those seeking to circumvent laws banning the use of testosterone to enhance athletic ability or body building. If a law specifies testosterone, and you change the molecule just a little, it isn't testosterone any more even if it has the same effects.

Our only real interest in this book is the naturally occurring hormone, testosterone. Testosterone is recognized as the <u>male</u> steroid hormone because it stimulates body growth, strength, hair growth, and male sex organs. In a similar way the steroid hormones estrogen and progesterone are known as <u>female</u> hormones because of their role in the menstrual cycle and pregnancy.

Testosterone, while fundamental for sex and reproduction, is not necessary for life in the manner of cortisone. Quite the opposite of cortisone, it is anabolic (biologically constructive). Testosterone has a powerful effect to build up and strengthen the body. Among other things it makes bones and muscles stronger and larger, and stimulates the bone marrow to make more red blood cells which carry oxygen to the tissues.

Testosterone is made in large amounts in the testes and in much lesser amounts in the ovaries and even in the adrenal glands. The surge of testosterone and other hormone secretion at puberty leads to the rapid growth spurt at that age and sexual maturity in both sexes. The much greater amounts secreted by the testes is largely responsible for the larger size and greater strength of men.

Unfortunately, because of its powerful anabolic effect, testosterone and its synthetic relatives are illegally over-used in harmful amounts by many to enhance strength, muscular size, and athletic performance. This is a gross, dangerous, and unhealthy misuse of the hormone.

2

The Foundation For the Book

I began using testosterone replacement therapy over thirty years ago. Like all primary care physicians caring for adults I had a number of elderly female patients who still retained the mental ability to have a full and active life but didn't have the physical strength or stamina to live one. These women were imprisoned in their enfeebled bodies. I wondered then if testosterone, because of its effect to strengthen muscles and produce more red blood cells, would be of any benefit to them. Could it improve the lives of those having a body too weakened by age to do what their younger minds wanted to do? I began giving small doses of testosterone to women over seventy-five, women who had their full mental capacities and who understood what we were doing. It almost always worked wonders. These women began to feel much better, stronger, had a better frame of mind, and became much more active. They started going to shows again, shopping, even resuming housework. Many also reported, with some embarrassment, the re-appearance of sexual feelings. I can recall one little, frail, eighty-five year old, looking away at the ceiling and coloring as she said in her squeaky voice, "I never thought I'd feel that way again."

My other use of testosterone during those years was in those occasional men who spontaneously offered a complaint about their loss of libido (sexual desire). Like most practitioners do today I would check their serum testosterone level. If it came back below normal, which very few did, I would treat them with testosterone injections, usually with excellent results. If their testosterone levels came back within supposedly normal limits, which almost all did, I'd blame their sexual problem on some other cause, usually tension, anxiety, or stress. I was never comfortable with blaming their sexual problem on these psychological causes, but since at the time I had no reason to doubt the validity of the testosterone blood test reports, I had no alternative explanation.

My heightened interest in the possible consequences of testosterone deficiency began about eight or nine years ago when I was asked to see John C. in consultation for his anemia (low number of red blood cells). He was hospitalized for a lung infection but wasn't severely ill at the time. A fairly complete laboratory workup for anemia had been done by his primary care doctor but there wasn't a clue as to why this sixty-six year old man was so anemic. There was a wheelchair at his bedside, and when I asked him during the course of my history taking why he couldn't walk, he replied that he didn't know.

Obviously, that was a very surprising answer coming from a well educated, mentally alert, man. It turned out that John had seen numerous neurologists during the previous few years but no one had been able to tell him why, "I can't bear my weight," as he put it.

Assuming that no neurological disease would have escaped detection by a half-dozen neurologists, to me John's phrase implied that he was suffering from a severe muscular disease. Understand that while John's anemia was significant, it wasn't nearly severe enough to account for that degree of weakness. The only condition I could think of that could even theoretically connect such profound muscular weakness with his unusual, unexplained, anemia, was severe testosterone deficiency. Recall that testosterone has a major stimulating effect on the bone marrow to produce red blood cells.

As I stated, testosterone deficiency was only a theoretical consideration, certainly not a realistic possibility. I had never heard of testosterone deficiency causing this degree of anemia, nor had I ever heard of testosterone deficiency causing such severe muscle weakness. I asked many of my colleagues if they had ever heard of such a thing. They hadn't.

I really didn't believe at the time that it was possible for testosterone deficiency to be so profound that it would prevent a man from standing. Even when his testosterone level came back extremely low I still had major doubts as to any cause and effect relationship between the hormone and his weakness and anemia. I was completely wrong. Just a few months of testosterone injections resulted in him gradually regaining his strength, first to stand, and then to walk, ultimately with just a cane for support. His anemia in the meanwhile disappeared.

To me, my experience with John was astonishing. I was amazed to have learned just how profound the consequences of testosterone deficiency could be, and it put testosterone in the forefront of my mind.

With almost all diseases there is a broad spectrum of severity. One person can be at death's door from pneumonia while another just has a cough, feels fatigued for a while, but doesn't even miss work. With congestive heart failure, one person can be in pulmonary edema, near death, while another only notices some shortness of breath while carrying packages up stairs. A person with hypothyroidism (underactive thyroid) at one extreme can be in a coma, while others another only notice a bit of lethargy and some cold intolerance. As would be expected, with most diseases the more minor and moderate manifestations are far more common than the very severe. *After John C., what buzzed in the back of my mind was: If a major testosterone deficiency can be so devastating, where were all the milder problems caused by more moderate deficiencies?*

My first considerations, in view of the commonly appreciated nature of the hormone, were sexual. I began to wonder if those men who complained of loss of libido, but had low-normal testosterone levels, were really suffering from stress and anxiety. Could they actually be physiologically deficient in testosterone, and respond sexually to treatment with the hormone? I began to treat those men who had low-normal testosterone levels, and almost every one became interested in sex again. This was when I began to see and understand that the so-called "normal" laboratory values for testosterone weren't a reflection of reality. Very simply, they were, and are, wrong.

Up until this point I was involved only with those men who spontaneously vocalized a complaint about their loss of libido. I next began to wonder exactly how prevalent this problem of loss of sexuality was and began to ask, I mean *really* ask. The following is a make-believe conversation that would approximate a fairly typical examination room initial sex dialogue. My fictitious patient is Zeke.

"Having any sex problems?" I asked during the course of my routine questions.

Zeke smiled broadly, "No, everything's fine."

(Understand that Zeke has likely been a little jarred by the question because it is extremely unlikely that he had ever had a doctor ask him about his sex life before.)

"Just like when you were thirty?" I asked while putting on the blood pressure cuff, "Your libido is okay? You get horny?"

Zeke grew quiet. His smile faded. "No, not really."

"Most/many men your age," I said in the manner of informing him, "have very little sexual desire, or even none at all. Do you have any?"

"Not much," Zeke admitted.

"When was the last time you had sex?" I asked.

Zeke shrugged, "I don't know. Quite a while ago."

"Do you know why you lost your interest in sex?" I asked.

Zeke looked at me with expectant interest.

From the questioning of my patients I estimate that about four out of five men, or more, begin to lose their libido between the ages of forty-five and fifty-five, many even much younger. (There's a good probability that many of the others were lying.) Almost all of the men who were interested in regaining their libido, and took testosterone injections, did regain it and resume active sex lives.

It didn't take long for some guilt to creep into my soul. I was doing all this asking and discussing and treating for men, but not for women. I had long had the impression that many or most post- or peri-menopausal women had lost some of their interest in sex, but I really didn't know how common it was nor to what degree. Furthermore, based upon the sexual stimulation I had seen for decades in testosterone treated older women, it certainly seemed likely that if younger, peri-menopausal, women were having major loss of libido, testosterone injections should help them also.

After a prolonged period of self-castigation for not doing so, I finally summoned the courage and began to ask my female patients about their libido, their sexual activity, and their orgasms.

A lot of surprises were in store for me. After their initial shock and embarrassment, which rarely lasted very long, they almost all opened up, most happy and even relieved to do so. Many remarked that they had always wondered why their gynecologists never asked them about sex. It turned out that women's sexual problems were far worse than what I had been hearing from men. Not only did they have little, if any, sexual desire, as compared to what they had felt a decade or two earlier, but they also had dry vaginas, possibly painful intercourse, and found it difficult, if not impossible, to have orgasms. I began to give small doses of testosterone to those women who wanted to try it, and another of my many testosterone surprises was learning that sexual improvement from testosterone in the female is not only far greater than in the male, and not only occurs much faster than in the male, but also has many benefits unique to the gender that I did not suspect.

Many, many more surprises were in store for me. During the years that have followed my observations of replacement therapy in an expanding patient population uncovered many other, non-sexual, manifestations of testosterone deficiency. *I've come to the realization that physiologic deficiency of testosterone is a major, very common, unrecognized, disease state that is responsible for a multitude of serious adverse health issues.*

3

"Normal" Testosterone Laboratory Values

"Normal" and "Natural"

Before beginning the discussion about testosterone blood levels as determined by the usual tests for that hormone, it is important for the reader to first reconsider an almost universally accepted pair of impressions. For reasons that go far beyond the topic and scope of this book, people's minds have to be opened to a re-evaluation of their understanding and comprehension of two words. I am referring to the interpretation of the words, "normal", and, "natural". Both are routinely used in everyday conversation and advertising, but both are actually very complex, and very confusing, concepts.

Consider that "normal" means what is usual, what is average, what is <u>most common</u>. The word is also used to *imply* <u>good health</u>.

Consider that "natural" means the <u>conditions and consequences of nature</u> with the inference that it is unaffected by man's interference. This word is also used to describe many, many products in the health industry, always *implying* that they are <u>healthy</u>.

In the context that these two words are most often used they are grossly misleading because not only do they have no foundation in reality, but they are, for the most part, deceptive or illusional.

It seems that almost everyone has the reflexive perception that anything and everything labeled normal or natural must be good, safe, okay. In reality, not only is that not always the case, it's not even usually the case. What is normal or natural is more often than not very undesirable. The more that medical science has been successful, meaning the more that we've been able to interfere with nature and thwart or delay normal, natural, diseases and death, the more divorced from reality these two words have become.

(As a related side note, when it comes to "natural" plants and herbs, be aware that the U.S. Food and Drug Administration FDA poisonous plant database lists fifteen thousand and eighty-nine "natural" plants as <u>poisonous</u>. (That's: 15,089).)

When it comes to our lives:

> *There is nothing more normal and natural than disease and death. They are 100% certainties for all life forms.*

> It is natural and normal for us to develop higher levels of cholesterol and blood pressure as we age.

> It is natural and normal for our arteries to ultimately harden and clog and cause a stroke or a heart attack.

> It is natural and normal for our joints to steadily deteriorate and erode with age and cause us pain, disability, and incapacitation.

> It is natural and normal for our brains to slowly deteriorate and bring on dementia and senility.

> It is natural and normal for some cell in our body to eventually become malignant and become a fatal cancer.

> It is extremely natural and normal for some type of microorganism to take root in our body at some point, cause an infection, and kill us.

> It is natural and normal for us to lose our libido and become progressively weakened and enfeebled as we get older.

(If you think about it for a moment, every one of the above conditions is considered a disease except the last one.)

In summation, don't reflexively accept either of these two descriptive words as indicating or describing something desirable. When it comes to advertising I personally regard the use of the word, "natural", as nothing more than a catchword, a gimmick to lure the consumer into buying something that in all likelihood has little or no innate value. Always keep in mind that natural and normal things are sometimes good, and certainly very often beautiful, but more often the words are factually descriptive of disease, illness, and death.

LABORATORY DETERMINATION OF TESTOSTERONE LEVELS

Normal testosterone blood levels in this sense means the range of levels found in a large varied group of *presumed* healthy people. One of the current major problems with the diagnosis of testosterone deficiency is the past and present definition of "healthy". It keeps changing, and not only is the subject of continual disagreement, but, certainly, much historical error.

There are two common types of testosterone blood tests, the "total" and the "free". Free testosterone is the active hormone, the one that is actually doing something. Total testosterone includes the bulk of the hormone which is bound to protein in the blood and is inert, inactive. The experts at two major laboratories I use are both quite definite in their opinion that the free testosterone level is much the more important and accurate.

In the past, when blood tests for testosterone first became available, the ranges of normal had to be established. Thousands of "healthy" people were tested to determine the upper and lower limits of normal testosterone levels. For these people to be considered healthy they had to be free of disease—*as disease was defined*. No one was asked about their libido or their sex lives. Being chronically fatigued or mildly to moderately depressed was not a consideration. Osteoporosis in post-menopausal women was taken for granted. Severe weakening and debility of the aged was considered normal. I have presented this scenario of how normal levels of testosterone were initially determined to consultants at two major laboratories that I use, and both were in agreement.

The inadequate, deficient, blood levels of testosterone that I have come to believe are the cause of, or a major contributor to, many severe diseases have for the most part been labeled as being normal. The laboratories have unwittingly defined the hormone deficiency cause of these problems out of existence. (See the story of Al D. at the end of Chapter Five)

This blindness to a common disease state has simply perpetuated itself over the decades. If someone, (and it does not have to be someone old), chronically complains about unexplainable fatigue, for example, and their testosterone level is checked, *what could actually be a significant physiological deficiency will very possibly be within the listed normal range.*

The laboratories' definitions of normal testosterone levels actually lend support to my contention that the listed ranges are hiding deficiency states. One laboratory lists normal male free testosterone levels as being between 50 and 210. Another, using a different test method, lists .95 to 4.3 for adults under fifty, and .80 to 3.5 for adult males over fifty. (I don't accept older men having lower "normal" levels of testosterone just like I don't accept older men having higher normal levels of cholesterol, or higher normal blood pressure.) Notice that in all cases the upper limit of normal is more than four times the lower limit of normal. I've taken the normal limits for another active hormone, thyroid hormone, (T3), from several laboratories and averaged them. There is less than a two and a half fold difference between the upper and lower limits of normal.

If we raised the normal lower level of male free testosterone to reflect the same ratio as T3 we would have lower limits of normal around 90 instead of 50, and near 1.6 instead of .95. *By these numbers, 20% to 25% more testosterone test results would fall into the abnormally low or deficient range, and it's possible that percentage could be even higher.*

When it comes to women the evidence of the fallacy of currently accepted normal testosterone values is even more striking because the disparity is far greater. One laboratory lists normal female free testosterone values as being between 1 and 8.5. That's an eight hundred and fifty percent (850%) difference between two supposedly normal levels.

Another laboratory's normal free testosterone range for forty to fifty-nine year old women is .04 to 2.03. That's a fifty-fold difference between the low and the high. The human body simply doesn't work that way. Aside from pregnancy, two women can't have a five thousand percent (5,000%) difference in the quantity of an active hormone in their blood and yet both be healthy.

Two other laboratories actually have "0" (zero) as the lower limit of normal for free testosterone in women. In other words, these laboratories' values infer that testosterone deficiency does not exist in the female human being. According to these numbers, a woman can have no testosterone at all and supposedly be healthy. The irrationality of these definitions of what constitutes a normal range of free testosterone in the female is amply demonstrated by the fact that approximately half the testosterone in a woman is made in the adrenal glands, glands whose hormone secretions are essential for life.

Is it really possible that a major medical problem such as I propose, a hormone deficiency that is responsible for widespread disease, suffering, and death, can simply be unrecognized by the medical establishment in part because of incorrect laboratory values?

We can look at a very recent example of just such a phenomenon, a common, very serious, but unrecognized, disease state.

It wasn't very long ago that the accepted normal upper limit of the LDL (bad) cholesterol was 160. Then it was lowered to 130. Now, according to the government and major health organizations, the upper limit of acceptability is 100, and in some cases, 70.

What this means is that for many recent decades, everyone who had an LDL cholesterol between 100 and 160 had an unrecognized disease state, and a fatal one at that. I believe that the lower end of the accepted normal levels of testosterone in men and women is a similar unrecognized disease state.

In summation, in my opinion the currently accepted normal ranges of testosterone are erroneous, and paying heed to these values is one of the reasons the medical community is not recognizing what I believe are serious consequences of inadequate testosterone levels in all adult age groups. After years of observation I have set my own lower limits of normal or acceptability for testosterone, and it is significantly higher than the laboratories'. Treating people with these values with testosterone has almost always resulted in elimination or alleviation of the problem at hand.

4

Official FDA Approved Indications and Warnings

Hopefully, you now have some understanding of testosterone as a hormone and the problems with the laboratory determination of normal levels. It will be beneficial for the reader to have in mind the official FDA approved indications and warnings concerning the use of testosterone while considering my experiences, conclusions, and speculations. Be forewarned, it is very confusing.

FDA Indications (The Confusion and the Bias.)

The following is the *only* official indication for an injectable brand of testosterone. I have X'd out the brand part of the name.

"X Testosterone Injection is indicated for replacement therapy in the male in conditions associated with symptoms of deficiency or absence of endogenous testosterone."

("Endogenous" means the hormone that is produced by glands in the body.)

The FDA appears to have ignored approximately half the population, the female half. It certainly isn't an oversight on their part so there are only three possible explanations for their position.

1. It might be the FDA's judgment that there is no such thing as testosterone deficiency in the female.

2. It might be the FDA's judgment that there is such a condition as testosterone deficiency in the female, but they're not sure if it should be treated because there haven't been enough studies.

3. It might be the FDA's judgment that there is such a condition as testosterone deficiency in the female, but it simply shouldn't be treated.

Let's examine these possibilities.

They certainly can't hold to the first possibility, that there's no such thing as female testosterone deficiency, nor that it's not a disease. If a young woman has her testosterone secreting ovaries surgically removed, it must then, by definition, be followed by a testosterone deficiency state. This condition would have to come under the definition of being a disease just like every other hormone insufficiency resulting from surgical removal of the secreting gland(s). (In medical parlance it is common to use the prefix, "surgically induced", to more fully define the condition, such as surgically induced hypothyroidism if the thyroid gland is removed.)

In regard to the second possibility: Injectable testosterone has been available for at least fifty-three years. That's a very long time. Can it be that more than half a century hasn't been enough time to determine the efficacy and safety of testosterone replacement in surgically induced hypogonadism in the female? The lack of having answered these simple, basic, questions, issues that have been resolved for literally thousands of drugs during the past half-century, leads to the inescapable conclusion that the FDA's position is the third possibility. For some reason the FDA does not believe that testosterone deficient women should be treated.

Now matters start to become very confusing. The FDA approved official prescribing information specifies that the suggested dose of testosterone to be used:

"varies depending on the age, sex, and diagnosis of the individual patient."

(Did they stipulate, depending on "sex"?) There's more. The fourth of five FDA approved official contraindications is:

"4. Women who are or who may become pregnant."

(Did they say some specific "women"?)

Reasoning it out, the conclusion from the above is that there must be some reason, or reasons, for a woman to receive testosterone treatment, but having a deficiency of the hormone isn't one of them, and the FDA doesn't want to reveal what they are.

To add much more bewilderment, the FDA actually does officially approve some form of testosterone for use in women. The oral form of testosterone, which is actually methyltestosterone (methyltestosterone), combined in the same pill with an estrogen (female hormone) is officially approved to treat "a" menopausal symptom. Again, I have X'd out the brand names.

"X and X are indicated in the treatment of: Moderate to severe vasomotor symptoms associated with the menopause in those patients not improved by estrogens alone."

"Vasomotor symptoms" means flushing.

As I will mention again later, methyltestosterone, the oral form of testosterone, is less effective, and extremely more likely to cause liver problems, than the injectable form. *So while the less effective, more toxic, form of testosterone is approved for use in women, the more effective, non-toxic, form is not.*

Confusion reigns. By approving the use of methyltestosterone in women for menopausal flushing is the FDA inferring that this flushing is a symptom of testosterone deficiency? If that is the case then why is it approved only for this one single symptom of testosterone deficiency? And why isn't the safer, more effective, injectable form of the hormone approved?

Not only does the FDA's official policy on testosterone seem incomprehensible, but it appears to be an inescapable conclusion that the FDA is guilty of gender bias. They state that you can give testosterone to a male for, "symptoms of deficiency". That wording certainly permits a very broad scope of interpretation and opinion as to exactly what masculine complaints can be included in deficiency symptoms. Not much latitude is really needed, however, when it comes to libido. Loss of sexual desire is certainly one of the most common, and well recognized, symptoms of testosterone deficiency. You can, therefore, apparently among many other reasons, officially treat a man with testosterone in order for him to regain some of his lost lust.

The FDA doesn't officially permit such license with women, however. Their policy is to narrowly limit the use of the above-mentioned methyltestosterone—estrogen combination pill to only one specific feminine symptom of hormonal deficiency—flushing. In other words, while a man can officially use testosterone to get hot and have a good time, a woman can only use it to treat menopausal flushing. Doesn't seem very fair, does it?

The FDA's manifest confusion would appear to stem, at least in part, from a problem they have with coping with the existence of human sexual relations as a biological and physiological function. Considering the fact that testosterone is a primary and essential reproductive hormone, nowhere in these blurbs does the FDA address the connection between testosterone and the three-letter word they dare not mention. I'm referring to the one that begins with an "s" and ends with an "x". (No, not a baseball team and not a musical instrument.) In the real world that is the main reason that methyltestosterone-estrogen combination pill is prescribed. It behooves the FDA, or the powers that be over them, to discard their puritanical blinders and deal with the real world, to address the many physical, emotional, and sexual/social problems that result from testosterone deficiency.

FDA TESTOSTERONE WARNINGS (SCARE TACTICS?)

The following are the five warnings in the official FDA approved testosterone blurb: My comments are in italics below.

"Hypercalcemia may occur in immobilized patients. If this occurs, the drug should be discontinued."
No comment.

"Prolonged use of high doses of androgens (principally the 17 α alkyl-androgens) has been associated with development of hepatic adenomas, hepatocellular carcinoma, and peliosis hepatis—all potentially life-threatening complications."

The 17 alpha testosterone is the oral tablet form, methyltestoster-one. The injectable form is the 17 beta. I have never seen any liver problem from this.

"Geriatric patients treated with androgens may be at an increased risk of developing prostatic hypertrophy and prostatic carcinoma although conclusive evidence to support this concept is lacking."

Take note here of the strength of the official word that is used to connect testosterone to prostate cancer, it's a, "concept".

A full discussion of this warning, its profound effect on patients and physicians, and the relationship between testosterone and prostate cancer is presented in Chapter Eight

"Edema, with or without congestive heart failure, may be a serious complication in patients with pre-existing cardiac, renal or hepatic disease."

In over thirty years of using testosterone I have never seen it cause worsening of edema or congestive heart failure. I do believe, however, that there is an exceedingly important association between testosterone and congestive heart failure, again, in a quite different way, as is detailed in the heart failure section in Chapter Five.

"Gynecomastia may develop and occasionally persists in patients being treated for hypogonadism."

The relationship between gynecomastia (breast growth in the male) and testosterone is discussed in Chapter Five.

5

Non-Sexual Consequences of Testosterone Deficiency

OSTEOPOROSIS

Almost everyone is familiar with the problem of osteoporosis, a severe weakening of the bones that is a major cause of pain, disability, and even death in the elderly.

One very common misconception among patients should be addressed. Osteoporosis as such does not cause any pain or discomfort. The pain of osteoporosis comes when weakened bones are broken.

Everyone who is familiar with the concept of osteoporosis is probably also aware that it is far, far, more prevalent, and much more severe, in women. Almost no one who isn't a physician, however, really understands the basic nature of the disease, nor why it is such a greater problem in women. The public's lack of knowledge and understanding about the disease osteoporosis is not at all surprising. As unbelievable as it may sound, almost nothing they've ever seen, read, or heard, about osteoporosis is true. All the popular information media, and, unfortunately, most of the health and medical establishment also, have focused in on the *consequence* of osteoporosis, namely calcium deficiency, as if it was the cause. *There is no primary calcium deficiency state in osteoporosis. Calcium loss from the bones is the <u>result</u> of osteoporosis.*

In my book, "Get Well, Stay Well", published in 1988, I wrote the following:

"The physiologic and biochemical facts are that calcium can do little, if anything at all, for osteoporosis. The problem in osteoporosis is the loss of the protein matrix of the bone, the internal structure to which calcium adheres. Once this support is lost, the calcium disappears and will not be replaced no matter how much calcium is consumed. One normally builds a wall by first putting up wood studs, then nailing sheetrock or plasterboard to it. In this comparison the studs are the protein matrix of bone and the plasterboard is the calcium. If the plasterboard falls off, you can nail on a new piece. If termites have eaten the studs, however, you cannot nail plasterboard to air! The term fraud is not far from mind when you have a representative of a major pharmaceutical firm come into your office, ask you to recommend his brand of calcium, and then sheepishly apologize for talking about a treatment that everyone knows does nothing! I personally do not believe that a forced intake of calcium will have any beneficial effect on osteoporosis in an individual who has been on a reasonably balanced diet."

The above is nothing I discovered. It's what they taught in medical school a half-century ago! Bone is <u>not</u> a stable unchanging tissue. It is not like a brick. The internal protein structure of bone is constantly being eaten away by cells called osteoclasts while new protein matrices are being manufactured by other cells called osteoblasts. As the protein framework of the bone is disintegrating, the calcium is simply being washed away, ultimately out of the body into the urine. When new protein foundation is laid down calcium is taken from the blood and attached to it to make it strong.

Another analogy to bone would be reinforced concrete. When old iron reinforcing rods rust, the concrete surrounding them tends to crumble, and to a far greater degree than meets the eye. The serious deterioration and disintegration is occurring inside the structure, not just the cement crumbs that have fallen to the street or the sidewalk. When workers repair a decaying concrete structure they first lay down a new bed of crisscrossing reinforcing rods. Concrete trucks then appear to pour in the fresh concrete.

With bone, when the rate of construction falls behind the rate of destruction you develop osteoporosis and they break easily. When the rate of the internal destruction of concrete structures exceeds the rate of repair you wind up with bridges collapsing.

Information on the true nature of osteoporosis is readily available. A check of three online encyclopedias revealed the following descriptions of osteoporosis.

> … disorder in which the normal replenishment of old bone tissue is severely disrupted, resulting in weakened bones and increased risk of fracture;

> Thinning and weakening of bones because of a loss of tissue substance.

> … a disease of bone in which the bone mineral density (BMD) is reduced, bone microarchitecture is disrupted, and the amount and variety of non-collagenous proteins in bone is changed.

None of these encyclopedias state anything that could be interpreted as osteoporosis being a calcium deficiency disease. Bone "tissue", the word two of them use, does not mean just calcium. The third encyclopedia mentions protein, and rightly so, because it is elemental physiology that the calcium crystals in bone must be attached to protein.

I have never understood how this mass deception of the public began, nor why it has continued on for so long. Within the past year there was a well publicized report about a new study that confirmed what I learned during the early nineteen sixties, that taking calcium does not prevent or help osteoporosis. That report had no apparent impact on the public misconception of osteoporosis.

There actually does exist a condition where bones become weakened because of calcium deficiency. It's called "osteomalacia". Calcium and vitamin D intake cures <u>this</u> condition. For many decades it has seemed that the medical and pharmacological establishments have for some incomprehensible reason taken the definition and treatment of osteomalacia and applied it, unsuccessfully, to osteoporosis.

There are many common unhappy and tragic consequences of osteoporosis. One is thinning and weakening of the vertebral bodies, the bones of the spine. We all shrink with age due to compression of the intervertebral discs, the cushions between the vertebral bodies. Women, however, with their much more severe osteoporosis, are prone to vertebral body compression fractures. The bone scrunches, sort of like lightly stepping on a ping-pong ball. These fractures are very painful, even to the point of being severely debilitating, for about six weeks. I can recall one woman collapsing on the hood of a car. She was in so much pain she couldn't move. I have another memory of an older woman, who refused to go to a hospital, crawling out of my office on her hands and knees because she couldn't take the pain of standing.

Often these compression fractures primarily effect the front half of the vertebral bone, each scrunch causing a wedge shaped deformity which forces the upper body to bend forward a bit. There are a lot of vertebral bones that can scrunch, and with each there can be severe pain and an additional bending forward of the body.

Ribs are also severely affected by osteoporosis. Minimal pressure, such as leaning the chest on the rim of a bathtub while cleaning it, or even getting a somewhat enthusiastic hug, can break one or more of these bones. These fractures are also very painful and often lead to pneumonia because there's a tendency for affected women to breathe shallow and to try to hold back from coughing.

Fractured hips are another extremely common complication of osteoporosis, and the consequences are severe pain, hospitalization for surgery, further institutionalization for rehabilitation through physical therapy, or possibly becoming bed-ridden and suffering its attendant bed sores and recurrent pneumonia.

Now, why is it so bad in women? Remembering that testosterone has a marked strengthening effect on bone, is it merely a coincidence that women's levels of the hormone are not only much lower than men's when women are young, but lower to an even greater degree when women become older? If we look at the laboratory values in Chapter Three, the upper limits of testosterone, (what we have when we're young), are 210 for men and 8.5 for women. Young women, therefore, have about 4% of the testosterone of young men. The lower levels, (when we're old), are 50 for men and 1 for women. So older women have about 2% of the testosterone of older men. (And remember, many laboratories list 0 as the lower limit of female testosterone. [What this really means is that the quantity is too small to be measured.]) Is it any wonder that older women's bones are so easily breakable?

It is very likely that an inadequate blood level of active testosterone is the primary cause of osteoporosis in women, and since the only contraindications to the use of testosterone in women is advanced liver disease and pregnancy, there is no reason that this therapy shouldn't be initiated with the onset of menopause. Instead, the primary medical therapies now are either calcium and vitamin D, which do nothing, or medications which put a foreign chemical into women's bones to inhibit the osteoclastic cells that are destroying them. There have been some recent media reports of undesirable long-term consequences to this type of therapy. Wouldn't it make a lot more sense to correct the hormone deficiency that is causing the problem in the first place?

So, the next time you hear of a middle aged or older woman suffering with a fractured hip, or see an old woman with a dowager's hump, or so severely bent over that she can only see the ground at her feet, you are probably looking at someone with a severe, undiagnosed, untreated, testosterone deficiency, someone who has become deformed because of medical ignorance.

One final and very important word about calcium and vitamin D. While they do nothing to prevent or correct osteoporosis by themselves, once a woman begins to receive testosterone replacement these two nutrients become vital. The testosterone is stimulating new bone formation, and the body needs to have sufficient calcium to deposit in the new bone tissue.

MUSCULAR WEAKNESS AND ITS COMPLICATIONS

The profound muscle weakening (myasthenia) effect of extreme testosterone deficiency was brought sharply into focus by John C., (Also see the story of Al D. at the end of Chapter Five) but I've learned that even mild to moderate deficiencies can cause a significant loss of strength and easy fatigability in both sexes. It's common knowledge that both men and women get weaker as they grow older, and in all likelihood the major factor in that deterioration is their low levels of testosterone. If checked or questioned closely, most men and women in, or certainly past, their fifties will have some manifestations, some symptoms, of this deficiency. The onset of this weakness is so gradual, however, so insidious, that most people simply aren't fully aware that it's happening. They usually simply stop doing things they used to do because of the effort required, and so don't get a full appreciation of just how weak they've become.

I've noticed that when treating testosterone deficiency in men they often have no appreciation of their increased strength because they have stopped doing anything that requires that strength. When some circumstance arises that needs some significant muscle they then become aware of the change in their bodies.

One man who at first denied noticing any change in his strength, when asked to think about it for a moment realized that doing curls with the barbell in the gym had become much easier.

Another man was quite certain that the testosterone had done nothing for his strength. When I quickly went through a brief list of activities that require some effort he reacted to "climbing stairs". He and his wife had recently vacationed in Italy. He recalled that one day they wanted to visit an old historic church which required quite a hike up and over a large hill. The man had contemplated the hill with some dread, but had found the climb to be much easier than he had anticipated.

I've had two personal experiences with this phenomenon. My sailboat has a fairly high freeboard (the distance from the water to the deck), and I had found it very difficult to get aboard from a floating pier. I had to crawl on, knees first, or use a step stool I carried aboard. This had become my habit. Some several months after I began correcting my low testosterone level I had occasion to have to get aboard very quickly. The boat was blowing away from the dock! I grabbed the stanchions (railing posts) and just leaped up on deck. I stood there stupefied, amazed at what I had been able to do.

The autumn before I began testosterone replacement therapy I had found it impossible to pull some reinforced hoses off their hull fittings by hand. The boat mechanic who helps winterize my boat had to do it. To my amazement, the autumn after I began taking testosterone, I reached down, and with only moderate effort, yanked three hoses off, one right after the other.

Women who are treated for their testosterone deficiency are usually much more aware of their increasing strength. The change in females manifests itself more as a recharging of their energy levels rather than an increase in their ability to lift weights or do something else that requires greater strength. Almost all women report a greatly improved level of energy and stamina, a heightened sense of well-being. As will be discussed later, many women who have discontinued testosterone replacement for one reason or another come back to it because of the return of their chronic fatigue.

Testosterone replacement may very well be able to play a major role in improving the lives of the aged. Over the course of the decades I've seen many of my patients, still having excellent minds, be forced into nursing homes simply because they had lost the physical strength and stamina to care for themselves. I've not had the opportunity to study the effect of testosterone on many of these institutionalized older patients, although there is one case history in the next section. Patients of that age who are in my practice, however, show a significant and consistent improvement in their strength and energy when they receive testosterone.

Fanny T. is a ninety-two year old woman who has been my patient for decades. She is mostly confined to her home now, and I try to see her there as often as I can. Over the past many, many years I have been giving her small doses of testosterone, usually on a regular basis, sometimes not. The difference in the woman when I haven't seen her for a while, and she has lost the effect of the testosterone, is remarkable, as is the come back when renewed treatment has had its effect. The difference in her appearance, her movement ability and agility, even the strength and rapidity of her speech, is striking.

Testosterone has also had a marked effect on the life of Florence T. This tiny, frail, ninety-one year old woman has been getting small doses of testosterone for over four years. I initially began her on the injections because she was rapidily deteriorating, getting progressively weaker and more fatigued. Despite having an aide it was becoming apparent that being institutionalized was only a matter of months away. The testosterone resulted in a substantial improvement in her strength and energy to the point that she no longer had any difficulty living at home with her aide.

I had been wondering for a while if she might do better if we increased the frequency of her injections from every four weeks to every three weeks as we do with younger people. We began her on that schedule about six months ago, and there has been noticeable further improvement. Today, when she came to the office with her aide, I was told that she had taken a trip to Atlantic City the week before. Florence was very proud of her excursion and had enjoyed it immensely. When I asked her aide if Florence really had enough energy to do that sort of thing her reply was, "Are you kidding? She has more energy than me!"

There is little doubt but that Florence would have been in a nursing home for many years now without the strength and energy she gets from replacing her missing testosterone.

It might well be the case that routine replacement of depleted testosterone levels in the elderly could markedly reduce the population of nursing homes and assisted living facilities to the major benefit of the patients, their families, and the costs of caring for them.

Weakness that comes with older age can have, and does have, a profound adverse effect on the quality of people's lives, *but there is a lot more to the weak muscle story than just arms and legs. This testosterone deficient muscular weakness can manifest itself in some other, extremely important, ways.*

Respiratory Problems

You've probably have never given the matter much thought, but it takes a lot of muscular effort and energy to breathe, and especially to cough. One could even theorize that the muscular weakness that comes from testosterone deficiency could wreck havoc with the respiratory health of the older population. Indeed, I've come to recognize that testosterone deficiency is a prime cause of, or contributor to, many severe respiratory problems in the elderly.

There's a saying in medicine, "Old people die of pneumonia when they get too weak to cough." There's a lot of truth to it. In all of us, coughing is the reflex that prevents a routine chest cold from becoming pneumonia. Have you ever seen an older person, bedridden, trying with great difficulty to cough up some phlegm? It's a very common problem that essentially happens to everyone if they live long enough. There is an excellent likelihood that testosterone replacement therapy in elderly patients would increase their muscle strength to the point that coughing for them would become much easier and much more effective. The current incidence of pneumonia, and recurrent pneumonia, in the elderly could be dramatically reduced. Not only could many years be added to their lives, but many hospitalizations could be avoided. The cost of testosterone therapy for a year is less than the cost of staying in a hospital for two hours. The case history that follows shortly addresses this subject. As you will read, the results were not conclusive, but the change in the patient was profound.

That old medical saying should be changed to, "Old people die of pneumonia when their testosterone levels become so low that they're too weak to cough."

A lot of people hospitalized for severe heart or lung problems require intubation and mechanical ventilation. In other words, they have a tube inserted through their mouth into their throat and a machine does the breathing for them. Sometimes these people cannot be weaned off the breathing machine and a tracheostomy has to be done. (The breathing tube is inserted through a surgical hole in the trachea [windpipe] in the front of the neck.)

Often the patient cannot be weaned simply because of the advanced stage of their heart or lung disease, but sometimes it appears that the problem is not so much the severity of the heart or lung problem but rather the lack of sufficient strength to breathe. Because of the machines these people have not been using their respiratory (breathing) muscles to breathe for some time, and they have weakened from disuse. Add this newly acquired additional weakness on top of the significant weakening debility of testosterone deficiency in the elderly, and we have people doomed to have a machine breathe for them for the rest of their lives.

I had wondered for a long while if the muscular strength regained from testosterone administration would be enough to get some of these people breathing on their own again. I recently had an excellent opportunity to see and test a fairly typical patient.

Christine T. was eighty-eight years old when she developed pneumonia earlier this year. Despite her age, Mrs. T. was completely free of senility or dementia. She was an active housewife and mother, did the shopping for her family, and was interested in reading newspapers and watching T.V. Although I know this woman personally, and have provided some minimal medical care on a couple of occasions, my knowledge of this medical story comes primarily from multiple family members.

Mrs. T. was hospitalized for three to four weeks with severe bilateral pneumonia (both lungs) for which she had to be intubated (put on a breathing machine), and eventually have a tracheostomy. When the pneumonia finally did resolve she was unable to be weaned from the breathing machine. The family was told by the lung doctor that the problem was not due to advanced or continued lung disease but rather weak respiratory muscles. As explained above, Mrs. T. had not been using her breathing muscles all the while she was on mechanical ventilation and they had greatly weakened from simple lack of use.

Mrs. T. was transferred to a rehabilitation facility which cared for ventilated patients. After a stay of weeks they had no success in weaning her off the breathing machine.

After another brief hospitalization, Mrs. T. was transferred to an institute in another state which specializes in weaning patients off breathing machines. I was told that the medical staff there confirmed that Mrs. T.'s lungs were not her primary problem, but rather weak breathing muscles. This institution also had no significant success in their attempts to wean her. She became very short of breath as soon as the machine's breathing rate was turned down even a little.

I had been discussing the possible benefit of testosterone injections for Mrs. T. with her family. I told them that the testosterone might give her enough additional muscle strength to eventually get her off the breathing machine, and that there was really no downside to the hormone. They were all very much in favor of the idea. I wrote a letter to the physician in charge of Mrs. T. at that institution, and even included a prescription for a testosterone injection. They refused, dismissing the suggestion out of hand.

After a month of unsuccessful attempts to wean her, the staff at this institute ultimately came to the conclusion that Mrs. T. was simply not weanable. She was transferred to yet another rehabilitation facility which cared for ventilated patients near where we live. The family, and the patient, were very anxious for her to receive some testosterone as there was certainly no other hope of her ever getting off a breathing machine and coming home. The family received official permission from this facility for me to participate in her medical care.

On my first visit to Mrs. T. I found a woman who had gained about thirty pounds due to gross over-nutrition in the various institutions. (What a horrible thing to do to a person.) She had become very depressed, morose, disinterested in newspapers, T.V., even in communicating with her family. She had become too weak to even turn in bed without assistance. With her daughter's help I gave her an injection of testosterone.

I returned two weeks later. There hadn't been much change. Testosterone almost never does anything after only one injection.

I was told by family members that a few days after the second injection Mrs. T. suddenly began to perk up. She began moving in bed on her own, asked for T.V. and newspapers, and began actively communicating with her family by writing. As the days and next couple of weeks passed she made remarkable improvement in her breathing ability, so much so that her pleased and enthusiastic respiratory therapist was able to get her about halfway to being weaned off the machine completely.

At that point the Medical Director of the institution found out that I had been giving Mrs. T. testosterone injections, and for some reason became outraged. My treatment was no secret. I had written detailed progress notes in her chart, and had even written orders for the injections which I carried out myself. The man categorically refused to allow Mrs. T. to have any more testosterone injections in his institution. In writing he expressed his disinterest in whether the testosterone had had any beneficial effect, and made no effort at all to determine if my diagnosis of myasthenia (muscle weakness) due to testosterone deficiency was correct. He even threatened me should I go to his institution and give Mrs. T. another injection. I was, and remain, absolutely sickened and appalled.

I wrote him twice, informing him that he was discontinuing an established highly successful therapy, and that the patient's condition was soon going to deteriorate if the testosterone injections weren't resumed. They weren't. Mrs. T. has deteriorated. She relapsed into full requirement of the respiratory machine, has been hospitalized several times for pneumonia and other major problems. I've been told that she has undergone severe mental deterioration and is likely close to death. (Mrs. T. passed away during the early production phase of this book.)

I advise that anyone with a relative in this situation request that a trial of several injections of testosterone be given. Testosterone patches, creams, or pills, are not acceptable. In patients with an advanced stage of a serious illness there is certainly no downside.

Anyone who has watched those suffering from advanced chronic lung disease trying to breathe knows how much muscular effort it requires on their part. I haven't had the opportunity to evaluate such a patient with respect to testosterone deficiency and replacement, but having seen and experienced the marked strengthening effect of the hormone, I would be surprised if their lives weren't made much easier by being treated with it.

Congestive Heart Failure

Congestive heart failure (CHF) is an extremely common heart condition. It comes about when the heart has lost some of its effectiveness as a pump. Congestive heart failure is not in itself a disease. It is a condition, and is the consequence of some type of underlying heart disease. Regardless of the cause, the net result of congestive heart failure is the accumulation of salt and water in the body. This water settles either in the lungs causing shortness of breath, in the legs causing swelling (edema), or in both. The word "failure" has an ominous sound to it, as if death was something imminent, but that is not usually the case. People can go on for years, even decades, with congestive heart failure, if they take the proper care of the heart failure and the underlying disease causing it. The extreme form of congestive heart failure is called pulmonary edema, and that can quickly lead to death.

It will be worthwhile to the reader to briefly review the standard treatments for CHF before progressing to the subject of this book.

Sometimes the primary treatment for congestive heart failure is directed at the underlying heart disease itself. For example, CHF can be a consequence of coronary artery disease. The heart muscle is so weakened by an inadequate blood supply that it can't contract strongly enough to pump effectively. Often, one of several types of surgical procedures available to relieve the arterial obstruction can improve or cure the CHF. Another example would be CHF due to an obstructing or leaking heart valve. The valve either doesn't open all the way or doesn't close properly. Like any other type of pump with faulty valves, its efficiency in moving fluid is markedly reduced. Surgical correction of the valve defect cures the CHF.

More commonly, however, the patient's underlying heart disease has been treated to the fullest extent possible, and the treatment of CHF becomes aimed at helping the heart and kidneys get rid of the accumulated excess salt water. Sometimes the cause of, or a contributor to, the congestive heart failure is an abnormal heart rhythm, the heart is beating either too fast or too slow. Control of the heart rate in these cases is critical. Medication to slow a very rapid heartbeat, or a pacemaker to speed up an excessively slow heart rate, may cure the CHF. Drinking less fluid may seem to be a logical treatment, but it usually isn't very effective. Water goes where the salt is, so elimination of salt from the diet is obviously a first step. Diuretics (water pills) are an important medication for this condition, as are ACE inhibitors or ARBs (types of blood pressure medication). Some beta-blockers have also been shown to help congestive heart failure. Many patients used to take a form of digitalis such as digoxin which can help the heart beat more strongly and lead to an increased formation of urine. There are also new types of pacemakers that not only control the heart rate, but also help the heart to pump more effectively.

Now to testosterone. A few years ago I began to wonder if the myasthenia, (muscle weakness), of testosterone deficiency, which I had learned from John C. can be so profound, could also affect the heart. The heart, after all, is just a muscle, and not all that different from the other muscles in the body. The more I thought about it, the more there seemed to be no reason that the heart wouldn't also be affected by testosterone deficiency.

I had a collective memory of many patients I had seen through the decades, elderly patients who one day would complain of being weak, fatigued. The fatigue never lessened, and I could never find a cause. After a period of months or years of worsening weakness they would one day complain of shortness of breath. They were in congestive heart failure. Intensive medical testing and referral to cardiologists never revealed the cause of their worsening heart failure, and eventually they died. I wondered—could these people have had an unknown heart disease, one that would be called hypogonadic cardiomyopathy? (hypo gonadic = low testosterone, cardio myo pathy = heart muscle disease)

During this period of contemplation I asked three cardiologists if such a condition was known, or had ever been postulated. They all replied negatively, but were very interested, even intrigued, by the possibility.

I had a patient, Laura S., a delightfully feisty woman in her nineties who for years had required hospitalization every few weeks to months for congestive heart failure. We would admit her, dry her out with intravenous medication, then discharge her, only to have her soon return to the E.R. gasping for air. At home, under the supervision of her caring daughter(s), she was taking all the medication that existed, or that was possible for her to take, for her condition, but it could not prevent her from filling up with water.

I discussed my theory about testosterone and CHF with Laura and with her daughter. They both agreed that she should try the testosterone. From the time of her very first injection of testosterone in January 2005, Laura was not hospitalized again for CHF for fourteen months. Repeated questioning of her, her daughter, and her aide revealed no significant shortness of breath—no more than would be expected from her moderate chronic lung disease. Repeated outpatient chest X-rays during this period, done for the express purpose of looking for any signs of congestive heart failure, never revealed even a hint of it. When she was ultimately hospitalized fourteen months later with shortness of breath, it turned out that the primary problem was not her heart but terminal kidney failure. Not wanting to undergo dialysis, she passed away shortly thereafter.

It is very possible, even very likely, that many, most, or even almost all, patients in the geriatric age group who are suffering from congestive heart failure have as a primary cause, or contributing factor, the heart muscle weakness that comes from testosterone deficiency.

I have another patient of many years, Richard T., an elderly, learned, and vibrant, gentleman, free of any senility, who has advanced, but fairly stable, coronary artery disease. For many years he has suffered with predictable angina (chest pain/pressure) when he walks a short distance, or when he tries to have active sex (as opposed to passive sex). There is nothing more that can be done for Richard's heart disease. His cardiologists have even ruled out any further angiograms.

Well over a year ago Richard came to my office one day complaining of shortness of breath. This was the first time he had ever suffered from this. Physical examination and a chest X-ray clearly revealed that he was in congestive heart failure. He improved to a good degree on water pills, but was still symptomatic. We discussed my belief that a low testosterone level, which he had, could weaken heart muscle and bring on or worsen heart failure. We also discussed the facts that most physicians, and the FDA, believe that testosterone is contraindicated in patients with "serious cardiac disease." I told him that I had little doubt but that his cardiologists would advise him to not take the hormone. While we knew he had "significant" heart disease, neither one of us knew if it should be labeled "serious" in view of its long stability. Richard considered it all and decided he wanted to try a few testosterone injections. His response was quite remarkable. After two doses of testosterone he became totally free of any and all symptoms of congestive heart failure—like it had never existed.

Richard spends his winters in Florida. He had received perhaps a half-dozen or so doses of testosterone before he went down there last year, and, acting on the advice of one of his cardiologists, he discontinued taking testosterone.

When he returned north this past spring he didn't feel as well as he had the previous autumn. He was much more fatigued, had some shortness of breath, and just didn't feel as healthy. It was his offered opinion that his problem was probably due to his lack of testosterone. He was in a quandary. He really wanted to resume the testosterone treatment, but one of his cardiologists had recommended against it. I told him that I disagreed with his cardiologist, but perhaps the man had information or knowledge or experience beyond mine. My suggestion was that he speak with his cardiologist again, to get from him the detailed reason or reasons for his negative opinion, and then make up his own mind. Richard did exactly that.

Apparently, from what Richard told me, the cardiologist could not present a reason for his opinion. It was simply his feeling. Richard decided to resume testosterone treatment.

Many months have passed now. Richard feels much more energetic, has absolutely no shortness of breath, and recently told me that he was able to have active sex without any shortness of breath, or even any chest pain, for the first time in a long, long, time.

There is more to Richard's story in the chapter dealing with Diabetes.

Congestive heart failure can certainly exist without it being a patient's major complaint. Several of my patients who I have treated for testosterone deficiency, and whose primary complaints have been sexual disinterest or excessive fatigue, also ultimately revealed that they suffered from some shortness of breath on exertion. They knew that they became short of breath when walking a distance, or climbing stairs, or carrying heavy packages, but never bothered to tell their doctor about it—me. As will be seen in the three following case histories, testosterone injections not only relieved their primary complaints, but their shortness of breath disappeared as well.

Roy M. is a new patient, a sixty-eight year old gentleman who was begun on testosterone therapy primarily because of excessive and worsening fatigue and loss of libido. He was also started on high blood pressure medication at about the same time. During his initial visits he denied having any symptoms, and had no signs, of congestive heart failure.

During his last visit, when Roy told me that he was feeling a lot better, I asked him for details.

"I have a lot more energy. I couldn't walk a half block before without breathing hard. Now I can go a half-mile without any problem. I don't know if it was the testosterone, the blood pressure pills, or the weight loss."

I was surprised to hear about the change in his breathing ability because that problem had never been aired. The reason he hadn't mentioned it was because he hadn't recognized his "hard breathing" as a medical problem, having long assumed it was simply due to his weight.

Roy is significantly overweight. While his weight loss of nine pounds is an excellent start, and a credit to his motivation, I doubt that it is enough to account for such a major improvement in his exercise tolerance. His blood pressure treatment did not include a diuretic (water pill), so that also would not likely be a significant factor in his improvement.

I see Roy as an example of a medical condition that I have come to believe is very common—mild, unrecognized, unreported, congestive heart failure.

Martin H., a very alive and very active seventy-year-old Manhattan businessman, was beaming when I walked into the examining room recently. He had come for his fifth injection of testosterone. Before I had the chance to ask him anything he excitedly exploded with: "I walked *nine* blocks last week! *Nine* blocks!"

I really wasn't certain what he was talking about. After calming him down I got the details. It seems that for the past many years he had always become short of breath after walking about two city blocks, and had long been in the habit of routinely getting a cab if the distance he needed to go was any greater. One day the previous week, after a business meeting, he had another business appointment nine blocks away. When he came outside the hotel the weather was so nice, and he felt so energetic, that he decided to walk a little before getting a cab. It was only after his arrival at his destination that he realized, to his amazement and joy, that he had walked the entire distance without any shortness of breath at all. To put it mildly, he was ecstatic to be free of a long-standing symptom he had never reported to me.

Here again is a man who has had chronic symptoms of congestive heart failure, the condition coming on so gradually that it had become part of the routine of his life. Understand, I always ask about breathing during every checkup. There simply had never been a sudden enough change in Martin's breathing for him to think of mentioning it to his doctor.

Allen Y. is an eighty-four year old gentleman who had complained to me about his fatigue for quite a while. He was unhappy. It was obvious that he did not have the energy to live the life he was accustomed to and desired. When questioned, he did admit to some shortness of breath, but it wasn't a significant problem.

Allen's testosterone level came back low. We discussed testosterone and the fact that many doctors believed it could cause prostate cancer. I told him that I did not believe that was the case, but that many men his age could have early or hidden prostate cancer, and testosterone would likely stimulate its growth. I also told him that if that happened, the commonly used anti-testosterone drugs would likely stop its growth. Allen was really unhappy with the way he was feeling and really wanted to try the testosterone.

It wasn't long before Allen was coming to the office with a big smile and a sparkle in his eye. He had a very dapper side to his personality that I hadn't known about before. He told me that he was feeling a lot stronger, had a great appetite, and had also had some sexual feelings he was happy with. I wanted to know if he had noticed any change in his breathing, and we had the following dialogue.

"Does your breathing feel any better since you've been taking the shots?" I asked.

"Oh, yeah," Allen replied with an emphatic nod, "A lot. I used to have to stop after one block."

"And now?"

"I just keep walking."

I wanted more clarity to exactly how much of a change he had experienced. "Do you have less shortness of breath," I asked, "Or none at all?"

"None. I just keep walking."

I still wanted to find out if there was some limit to his improvement. "How far?"

Allen thought for a moment then shrugged, "I just keep walking."

"And you're stronger?"

"Oh yeah," Allen replied with conviction, "A lot stronger. I used to use the banister to pull myself up the stairs. Now I just walk up."

Here again is an elderly man with years of symptoms of congestive hear failure that had been mild enough to be ignored, but disappeared with testosterone therapy.

These three gentlemen, along with many thousands, perhaps even hundreds of thousands, of others likely have the heart disease I postulated earlier, hypogonadic cardiomyopathy. Over many years their heart muscle had become gradually and progressively weakened by a declining, inadequate, amount of testosterone. The resulting congestive heart failure had come on very, very, gradually, the men adapting to it by controlling their activity to minimize any breathing discomfort. Testosterone replacement had relatively quickly restored strength to their hearts, and the degree of their congestive heart failure problem became far more noticeable because of the rapidity of its disappearance.

In summary, *testosterone deficiency is likely to be a fairly common cause of, or contributor to, many cases of congestive heart failure. If heart muscle has become weakened by low testosterone levels, and the administration of that hormone strengthens it even a little, there could be a major improvement in the severity and symptoms of the heart failure. I recommend that anyone in chronic, or refractory, or severe, congestive heart failure be given a several month trial of testosterone injections. Testosterone patches, creams, or pills, are not acceptable. Unless the patient has prostate cancer, there is no likely downside. In my experience the reported potential of the hormone to retain salt and water has not been a clinical factor.*

PSYCHIATRIC

Timidity and Anxiety

I've seen a fairly consistent effect of testosterone therapy on fearfulness or timidity in both sexes, and from both perspectives. Many women have reported that testosterone makes them a bit more aggressive, and not only in the sexual sense. Perhaps, "assertive", is a better word. One male colleague who is a friend of a female patient of mine, and who knows about her testosterone replacement therapy, once jokingly asked me to reduce her dosage because of her heightened assertiveness at work.

On the male side I've seen a lessening of a vague feeling of fearfulness after initiating testosterone therapy. The well-known fearlessness of male youth is likely related to high testosterone levels. Eighteen to twenty-two year olds make the best, bravest, soldiers. As I mention later in the book, in the animal world testosterone seems to have a profound effect to enhance physical aggressiveness. Since anxiety is a quality of fear, I've wondered if testosterone would have any effect on chronic anxiety syndromes. I recently asked this question of one of my male patients in his late fifties. In the past he had suffered from anxiety, even panic attacks, had consulted psychiatrists, and had taken anti-depressants and tranquilizers. His response to my question was that, although he didn't know if the testosterone injections were the reason, he's had no significant anxiety since starting the hormone therapy. (Also see the story of Al D. at the end of Chapter Five)

<u>Depression</u>

Through the years I've seen a frequent, even consistent, elimination or lessening of depression as a result of testosterone injections. I am not for a moment suggesting that testosterone deficiency is a major cause of depression, but it could be the cause in some, and a significant contributing factor in many others. The only way to know is to check the free testosterone level and initiate a trial of therapy.

I have a patient whose rather severe, prolonged, depression and fearfulness appears to have been primarily due to testosterone deficiency.

Bruce R. is a single man in his forties who was suffering for many years with progressive depression, lassitude, and non-motivation. He had long lost his interest in sex, and had a failing relationship with his girlfriend. Every time I saw him he seemed to be more and more disinterested in life. He kept gaining weight, became progressively less talkative, and at one point began to become fearful. He even became afraid to drive the common vehicle that was his livelihood. Various antidepressant medications during these years had done very little. Prior to my considering that he might be suffering from testosterone deficiency, Bruce had arrived at a point of having lost his job and having no desire to do anything. He wasn't suicidal, but he honestly didn't care if he lived or died. I checked his free serum testosterone level. It came back very low, and we began a trial of therapy.

Nothing changed significantly after three doses of testosterone. We were both on the verge of giving it up. After the fourth injection, however, there was a profound change. Bruce became animated, talkative. He told me of the plans he was making for his future, and that he had become interested in sex again. His relationship with his girlfriend was revitalized. He was actually smiling! The change in him was absolutely amazing, and has continued. When he comes in for his shots I get the sense of a man who feels he's been reborn.

In cases of refractory depression in the appropriate clinical setting, and if free testosterone levels on the low side support the possibility, I believe a trial of testosterone is warranted. Once again, I would only suggest intramuscular injections, and given my above experience, at least a four to five month trial.

A couple of women I've had the opportunity to follow closely have had interesting fluctuations in their emotions that seem to depend upon the time of their testosterone month.

Joan H. at fifty-eight has a very strong character and stable personality, the rock of her family. She rarely experiences, or at least displays, any anxiety or depression, at least not during the approximately six years she's been getting small doses of testosterone replacement therapy. She's been getting her injections exactly every three weeks for years, but recently had a four-week gap. On the day she came in for her injection she had complaints that were unusual for her. She had suffered from nocturnal palpitations three nights in a row, was nervous, jumpy, and had several episodes of flushing and sweating.

I suggested a cardiac event monitor to learn the nature of her sudden palpitations. She wanted to wait and see if they continued. I drew blood tests to see if there was anything there that would give us a clue as to what was wrong.

As it turned out all her symptoms completely and permanently disappeared within about twenty-four hours of the testosterone injection. It hadn't occurred to either one of us that her symptoms might have been due to testosterone insufficiency. We decided to see what would happen after another four week interval. On day twenty-four she came to me with complaints of not feeling well, of being nervous and anxious and very short of breath at times. Once again all these symptoms disappeared by the day after the injection.

Cheryl R. is fifty-two years old and has been troubled with varying degrees of anxiety and depression all her life. She began testosterone injections for a failing libido almost two years ago, stopped for about eight months because of facial hair, then resumed treatment six months ago. More recently she took two consecutive very small doses because of her fear of a possible reappearance of facial hair.

When she came in for her next injection she complained of being excessively anxious, very depressed, tired, and in general "felt lousy." She also hadn't felt like having sex since the previous testosterone injection three weeks earlier.

We both had the time to discuss her moods and libido in relation to each other and to her testosterone injections. She easily recalled that months earlier, when she was getting a higher dose of testosterone, she was very libidinous, having relations with her husband about three times a week. She also felt very calm and free of depression at that time. She wasn't even experiencing much anxiety despite the fact that a major family affair was only a couple of weeks away. As she thought about her emotions and libido during the time she had been taking testosterone it seemed that for the most part, the more she was desirous of having sex, the less depressed and anxious she was.

There is no postulation here that having sex cures depression and anxiety, but rather that there is no doubt but that testosterone exerts significant effects on the mind as well as the body. These two women are further evidence that testosterone deficiency should be investigated as a possible contributing factor in all cases of chronic anxiety or depression.

VAGINITIS

Vaginal discomfort and irritation is not an uncommon problem, and sometimes it is resistant to usual modes of therapy. To my surprise, a number of women of various ages have told me that their chronic or recurrent vaginal irritation disappeared after they started taking testosterone.

Celia R. was in her early seventies when we first discussed testosterone about two years ago. She's a very attractive and young at heart woman who was unhappy with the effects of aging, with the loss of her love life and her worsening fatigue. She tired easily and was somewhat depressed. Celia is an unusual patient in that it was she who broached the subject of testosterone. While most men are readily agreeable to discuss testosterone and undergo a trial of therapy, women are usually much less so. In the case of Celia, her peri-menopausal daughter was receiving testosterone replacement therapy from me for sexual reasons, with excellent results, and Celia was interested to know if the shots might also help her. She and her long-term companion, Harry R., hadn't had any libido or sexual relations, for many, many years. As a matter of fact, she hadn't even thought about sex for a decade.

Celia had also been suffering from an intermittent, frequent, mild, vaginal itch and discomfort for about twenty years. When we began her treatment I purposefully did not mention that I thought the testosterone might also help her vaginal problem. I didn't want to raise hopes or expectations and have her be disappointed.

After about a year of therapy, when the sexual, energizing, and strengthening benefits of the shots were obvious, ongoing, and had become routine, I remembered her recurrent vaginal discomfort and asked her about it. She looked at me with a smile of surprise on her face, "You know, I forgot about that!" she said, very pleased that it had disappeared, "I haven't had that for a long time!"

The following story is especially striking because of the horrendous severity and longevity of the vaginitis, and the truly unbelievable rapidity with which it completely disappeared.

Evelyn I. is now fifty-three years old. At the age of thirty-five she developed vulvovaginitis. ([vulvo—vaginitis] The vulva is the external part of the female genitalia. The vagina is actually the canal inside.) That was the beginning of seventeen continuous years of relentless, constant, severe, genital inflammation. She describes sex as having been intolerable, impossible to bear. "I was so red and inflamed and swollen that sometimes I would go to bed with an ice pack between my legs." During these seventeen years she consulted many different gynecologists including those who were specialists in her type of problem. None of their various treatments were effective. She was told that she had vulvadynia, a simple, descriptive, diagnosis meaning vulva pain. Inherent in a purely descriptive diagnosis like this is the understanding that the actual cause of the affliction is unknown.

Evelyn joined the National Vulvadynia Association and was a support group leader there for many years. Her chronic inflammation was so severe that four years ago she had a pre-malignant skin lesion removed from a vaginal lip. The problem also affected her urethra, (the tube from the urinary bladder to the outside). It was so contracted and narrowed from the chronic inflammation and scarring that the flow of her urine was obstructed. She had been seeing a urologist regularly for the past four years. Every two months he would use a probe to stretch open her urethra so the urine could come out more freely, a procedure called urethral dilatation.

For several years I repeatedly suggested that she try a few testosterone injections. Based on my previous experience with much milder vaginal problems, I thought there might be some chance the hormone would help her. There was really nothing to lose by trying a few doses. Every time I suggested it, however, she'd consult a gynecologist who would advise her that testosterone wouldn't help and not to take it. I decided to do a free testosterone blood test on her. Perhaps that would persuade her. It came back at a level within the laboratory's normal limits but below my acceptable level. After I literally begged her, she finally agreed to try a couple of injections.

This is where Evelyn's story gets unbelievable. She walked into my office five days after the first injection and told me that 80% of her inflammation and pain were gone. She had even had sex the night before with minimal discomfort. About a week after the second injection she was completely symptom free. To be certain that she wasn't just fooling herself she decided to consult a new gynecologist and get a fresh, unbiased, opinion. She was told that there was nothing wrong with her, everything was normal. As some time passed her urologist told her that her urethral problem seemed to be getting a lot better. She later revisited her former gynecologist who was amazed to see that her vaginitis was gone and even questioned her about what she had done to clear it up.

The cause and effect relationship in this case, that her vaginal disease was caused by testosterone deficiency and that the administration of the hormone eliminated it, is an absolute certainty. Evelyn has had a few, very minimal, relapses of the vaginitis occurring around the nineteenth to twenty-first day after an injection, a time when the hormone level in her body has dropped below a sufficient level. Another injection of testosterone at these times always results in her minimal vaginitis quickly disappearing, usually in less than a day. There is no doubt but that this woman's long standing, severe, vaginitis was the direct consequence of the disease of testosterone deficiency, and was cured by replacement therapy.

Needless to say, keeping in mind that pregnancy is an absolute contraindication to testosterone therapy, (The hormone can sexually deform a fetus.), a free testosterone blood test and a trial of a few doses of the hormone should be given to women suffering from chronic refractory vaginitis, or who have been diagnosed with vulvodynia. Again, testosterone patches, creams, or pills, in my opinion, are not reliable enough to be used in a therapeutic trial.

Evelyn's chronic vaginal problem was labeled vulvodynia because the underlying cause was not known. There are many women, however, in whom the cause is known, at lease to some degree. I'm referring to women with chronic or recurrent vaginal infections. We are not including STD's (sexually transmitted diseases) in this discussion. Bacterial vaginosis is a bacterial infection of the vagina, and moniliasis or candidiasis is a yeast infection. Many women are familiar with the latter because that's the vaginal problem often brought on by the taking of antibiotics. Uncontrolled or poorly controlled diabetes also predisposes to vaginal yeast infections.

A healthy vagina is one that maintains the ideal chemical environment for the growth of good bacteria. Lactobacillus is the name of the organism that normally inhabits the vagina. Its presence in large numbers inhibits or prevents the growth of unwanted microorganisms. It does not require a great stretch of the imagination to wonder if hormone levels, especially testosterone levels, have an effect on the vagina's chemical milieu and bacterial population. It would be appropriate, therefore, that a trial of testosterone therapy be undertaken in cases of recurrent vaginal infection because it's quite possible that a deficiency in the hormone might alter the vaginal environment in a way to predispose to infection.

<u>FATIGUE</u>

Excessive chronic fatigue has been either the primary or secondary complaint for almost all of my patients whom I have treated with testosterone. There is no question but that low testosterone levels result in fatigue, but think about this: *Every medical condition that brings about excessive fatigue is recognized as a disease, and is evaluated and treated as such, except testosterone deficiency. It is an absurd, twisted, and illogical mind-set to perpetuate a willful blind eye to a symptom producing hormone deficiency.*

Chronic fatigue is such a common accompaniment of testosterone deficiency, and is relieved so readily, that other than one case where the fatigue was severe and compelling (see Chronic Fatigue Syndrome), there was no reason to include any specific case histories. Almost every patient reported here complained of fatigue to some degree. I have, however, included some case histories of the phenomenon of "unnoticed" improvement in fatigue.

Over the years I've seen that some patients on testosterone therapy experience significant improvement in their overall sense of well-being, but don't realize it. The effect of the hormone replacement sneaks up on them without them being aware. It is not uncommon, and happens to both men and women.

Larry D. is an eighty-two year old gentleman who is an excellent example of this phenomenon. A widower who lives in an assisted living residence, he had long complained to me about his fatigue. We discussed testosterone replacement therapy a few times, and eventually, despite some misgivings, he decided to try it.

During the early spring of 2006 Larry received four injections. He never noticed any difference in the way he felt. While he did look more lively, more animated, and less fatigued, to me, he was quite definite and certain that nothing had changed. We discontinued the treatment in May.

During the first week of July Larry came in for a routine checkup. The first words out of his mouth after our greetings were, "I want those shots again." Larry had returned to his chronically fatigued state, wasn't doing much, and realized how much better he had felt on the testosterone therapy. Now, two and a half months later, after four doses, he's going to Manhattan and Atlantic City regularly, walks faster, has lost all his shortness of breath, and enjoys people telling him how good he looks.

Retrospectively, it may be the case that because of his concerns Larry unconsciously didn't want to feel better from the testosterone. Those concerns, however, turned out to be no match for the feeling of good health that comes from eliminating a debilitating disease.

Doris M. was fifty-two years old when she was questioned a couple of years ago and admitted to a libido that could use substantial help. She's a very attractive woman and was actively dating at the time. She thought it would be great to actually want to have sex with her man. The testosterone injections certainly did that for her. She began to look forward to her evenings and the experience of sexual satisfaction.

After a time, however, Doris apparently became a little disgusted with the quality of the men in her life and decided to abandon the dating scene. She stopped taking her testosterone shots, reasoning that there was no point in promoting sexual needs when she was going to live a single life.

A few months later Doris was back in my office because she didn't feel very well. She was chronically tired and depressed. The energy and frame of mind she had enjoyed while taking the testosterone was missing. She just hadn't realized, or even noticed, how much the hormone had improved the non-sexual part of her life. Unfortunately for Doris at that time, *all* the symptoms of a hormone deficiency are alleviated by replacing the hormone. She vacillated for quite a while, taking a few shots, then stopping again, trying to recapture her sense of physical and mental well being while not stimulating any sexual needs. She wasn't able to have it both ways.

There is a happy ending to this story. Doris finally met someone she felt was suitable for a long-term relationship, and she wanted everything the testosterone did for her.

David G. is a sixty-two year old man who came to suddenly realize by himself the energizing effects of testosterone replacement. He began the hormone injections to see if it would really help his failing libido as I claimed it would. The trial of therapy was very successful. I usually question my patients if they've experienced any other effect of the hormone besides alleviating the primary problem. After several injections Dave told me that he had a much stronger libido, and much more intense orgasms, but hadn't noticed anything else.

A month or so later, during his last visit, Dave told me that he had recently had a revelation. He had been puzzled for several months over why he felt so much stronger and energetic. He felt extraordinarily full of energy in the morning, and then felt "vibrant" all day. For years he had been in the habit of taking an afternoon nap. Now he "keeps going all day and doesn't get tired until bedtime". It was only a week earlier that it had finally dawned on him that he was feeling a non-sexual effect of the testosterone.

David had certainly experienced the energizing effects of testosterone when I had asked him a couple of months earlier. Focused on the substantial sexual improvement, however, he hadn't connected the hormone with his sudden "vibrance".

These cases simply point out that there is more to a trial of therapy with testosterone than just asking the patient if he feels any better while taking it. Sometimes it's even more important to find out if the patient feels any worse when he stops taking it.

The positive response to the testosterone in alleviating fatigue has certainly well exceeded 90%. That degree of effectiveness certainly brings us to wonder about the possibility of there being a testosterone deficiency association with the so-called, Chronic Fatigue Syndrome.

Chronic Fatigue Syndrome

Prior to quite recently I was never convinced that a Chronic Fatigue Syndrome really existed. (All that business years ago about the syndrome being caused by Epstein Barr virus antibodies was and is pure nonsense.) Now, however, I'm not so certain. Perhaps a Chronic Fatigue Syndrome does exist.

Sarah E. is a forty-three year old divorced mother who has been a patient of mine for about six years. She has a busy life, works full time, has a close and intimate relationship with a male partner, and, interestingly, had a healthy and active libido before beginning testosterone injections.

After over two years of seeing her for routine checkups during which she had essentially no medical symptoms, she one day complained to me about being unusually tired and fatigued. This became a major negative factor in Sarah's life, an ongoing, daily, problem that she complained about during every visit to me for the next two to three years.

"I can't get out of bed in the morning."

"When I get home from work I just fall into bed. I'm too tired to do anything."

Repeated medical workups revealed no abnormalities. I could not, and would not, attribute her fatigue to stress or anxiety. It had come on too abruptly and was out of character. Since she had no sexual dysfunction I doubted that testosterone deficiency was playing any role in her problem, but eventually, out of frustration, and after discussing it with her, we decided to check her level. It came back in the range I consider to be inadequate. We both wanted her to try a few shots.

Sarah had no reaction to the first injection. When she returned for her third dose, however, she related that when she awoke on the third morning after the second injection she, "... knew that something had drastically changed as soon as I opened my eyes." She jumped out of bed. She felt like a new woman, almost a different person. Her chronic fatigue and tiredness were simply gone. The shots had also had an effect on her libido, and she laughingly described frequently pulling her boyfriend into bed. She was obviously over stimulated. A dose reduction solved that problem, but her fatigue and tiredness remained, and continues to remain, a part of her past.

Every adult person complaining of chronic fatigue, regardless of age or sex, and whose medical workup for that problem has been unfruitful, should have a free testosterone blood level done. Keeping in mind the danger of pregnancy, if the free testosterone level is below normal, or in the bottom 40% of currently accepted normal values, a trial of injected testosterone is warranted.

ANEMIA

Mild anemia is a very common accompaniment of old age, especially in women. While older people are commonly victims of diseases that bring on anemia, testosterone deficiency by itself has historically been a known cause. Unlike my experience with John C., anemia of testosterone deficiency is usually mild to moderate. The existence of the condition, however, is important for two reasons.

Firstly, *despite prevailing medical opinion, I have long believed that mild anemia is a significantly debilitating condition in the elderly.* A young woman's normal Hct., (a measure of red blood cells), can vary from approximately 38% to 48%, the exact range depending upon how the test is done. Let's take an average figure of 43%. Now she has become old, frail, weak, and her Hct. Is 32%. This is a degree of anemia that would be ignored by the medical community. It would be considered an acceptable test result in a nursing home and probably not be treated.

It is, however, a 26% reduction in her red blood cells, a 26% reduction in the amount of oxygen delivered to her tissues. This oxygen is needed to provide muscle cells, including heart muscle cells, with energy. This oxygen is needed by the cells of the immune system to fight infection, and by white blood cells to eat germs. It is desperately needed by cells that are trying to repair something, such as a broken hip or a bedsore. A healthy young person can, <u>over time</u>, easily adapt to this degree of anemia, but in the elderly it might have serious, continuing, adverse health consequences.

There is another way to look at the significance of this degree of anemia. If a healthy young man were to have his Hct. drop from 43% to 32% over a short period of time, say a couple of weeks, he would become profoundly symptomatic and severely weakened. Needless to say, the fact that testosterone in the elderly strengthens the body *and* raises the Hct. is, in my opinion, a doubled reason for its use.

The second reason anemia caused by testosterone deficiency is important is simply that the very existence of the anemia is proof that testosterone deficiency exists as a disease. *As is the situation with excessive fatigue, there is no other condition than can cause anemia that is not considered a disease.* If any young person presented in a physician's office and was found to have a Hct. of 32%, it would be considered to be abnormal, the result of some disease, and that disease would be actively sought out. But if an otherwise healthy old person has a Hct. of 32% it is not considered to be abnormal or the result of a disease, even though they need the red blood cells more than the young. In my opinion this prevalent attitude is age discrimination and poor medical care.

Iron Absorption

As stated previously, it has been well known for many decades that testosterone and testosterone derivatives stimulate red blood cell production in the bone marrow. Since it's usually the case that Mother Nature does common sense things, that she usually does a complete job, I began to wonder if the hormone might also have an effect to increase iron absorption. It seemed reasonable that if the hormone was going to increase red cell production, it would also increase whatever was needed to effect that result.

Carol N. is forty-eight years old and has been my patient for a long time. I've known about her iron deficiency since 1995 when I did her first serum iron test. Despite ongoing oral iron therapy, every iron and ferritin test done during this eleven-year period has been either low or very low. For those of you who like to see numbers: (October 2005: iron = 20, ferritin = 2). She's been on consistent, and very successful, testosterone therapy for a prior poor to absent libido for over a year. Although she hadn't taken her iron pills for two months before her most recent blood test, her iron and ferritin levels came back within normal limits for the first time. (August 2006: iron =120, ferritin =16)

This is only one case, and it proves nothing, but this possible effect of testosterone on iron absorption deserves further investigation because many women during their menstrual years suffer from chronic iron deficiency even though the amount of their menstrual bleeding does not seem excessive. It might possibly be that these women are living with low testosterone levels.

DIABETES (TYPE TWO—ADULT ONSET)

I originally was going to briefly speculate on a relationship between testosterone and adult onset diabetes, and place it in the miscellaneous chapter near the end of the book. I have very recently learned, however, within the past days, that there are controlled studies that have established a definite connection between testosterone deficiency and type II diabetes.

The likelihood of there being some association between the two could have been inferred for quite some time. Consider the following.

Type II diabetes has been shown to be intimately involved with excess abdominal fat and a biochemical defect at the level of muscle cell membranes.

Large therapeutic doses of <u>cortisone</u>, which always worsens diabetes and may actually bring it on, markedly promotes truncal and abdominal fat, and significantly weakens muscle cells.

<u>Testosterone</u> markedly strengthens muscle cells, and probably reduces abdominal fat.

I've underlined three words/phrases above, and the statements about them have some words in common. Fat and muscle appear in all three, diabetes in only two. What is missing is the connection between diabetes and testosterone. Is there a connection here? It would be logical to suspect that testosterone would have a beneficial effect on the membrane defect found in type II diabetes, and, indeed, that has been found.

Harry S. is a gentleman in his seventies. He was started on testosterone replacement because of his totally lost libido. That part of his story appears in that chapter. What interests us in this chapter is that after almost a year on successful testosterone replacement therapy he seemed to have a relapse, the only patient of mine to appear to lose the beneficial effects of testosterone therapy. Harry didn't become ill, and he didn't really feel bad, he had just lost most of the substantial libido, energy, and vigor he had regained from the testosterone injections. He stopped taking a long walk every day. His sexuality disappeared. A relative told me that he had become more inclined to take a nap than to do something active. Repeated blood tests revealed nothing. Shortening the interval between injections did nothing. I was really puzzled. After a few months of this lethargy I decided there had to be something I was overlooking.

Harry has adult onset diabetes for which he had long been taking a single oral medication, one which does not commonly cause low sugar reactions. When he mentioned to me that he usually felt especially fatigued a few hours after breakfast, I wondered if a mild, lingering, hypoglycemia (low blood sugar) could be the cause of his energy loss. I told him to stop taking that medication for a while.

He called me back a few days later. I knew I had solved the problem just from the sound of his voice. "Doc! You got it!" Harry had become rejuvenated again.

In all likelihood the testosterone injections had significantly improved Harry's glucose metabolism, probably by some effect on muscle cell membranes, and the result was that his minimal diabetic medication had become an overdose.

One patient doesn't prove much. The next patient I saw who had diabetes and was also on testosterone therapy was Mary M., a woman in her fifties. She is a very informed and conscientious patient, and has had stable, well controlled, insulin dependent, type II, diabetes for many, many, years. She had been on testosterone replacement therapy for about one year. The hormone had restored her libido, her energy level, her self-confidence, and had greatly eased her depression.

In regard to her diabetes I asked Mary to think carefully. Had there been any change in the frequency of her hypoglycemic (low sugar) episodes since she began testosterone therapy? She replied without hesitation, "Oh, yes. I used to have one every month or two. Now I get it almost every week."

Here again we see an increased effectiveness of diabetic therapy. This change in the state of Mary's diabetes is likely due to the testosterone improving her sugar metabolism. It will be interesting to see if this beneficial hormonal effect on her diabetes will remain, fade away, or prove to be progressive.

The story of Richard T. was discussed in the section on congestive heart failure. Richard also has a very mild case of type II diabetes. He has never taken any medication for this condition.

HgbA1C (glycohemoglobin) is a blood test that tells doctors how well or how poorly diabetes is being controlled. A value under 6 is normal. If the number is under 7 or 7.5, the diabetes is considered to be well controlled. If it is over 8, the diabetes is poorly controlled.

Richard's HgbA1C after the first several months of testosterone injections, before he went to Florida, was 6.6. When he came north in April, after not taking testosterone for many months, the number had increased to 7. It is now September. He has been getting testosterone injections again for several months and his HgbA1C is 6.4. Again, there has been no direct treatment of his diabetes. It might be that these changing numbers reflect the beneficial effect of testosterone on type II diabetes.

Sam C. was the third diabetic patient getting testosterone injections who I checked. He is fifty-nine years old. For the past ten months he has been taking unchanging doses of an ultralong acting insulin along with three types of oral diabetic medication. He began testosterone replacement therapy about five months ago primarily because of a very poor libido. Sam checks his sugar level regularly. Prior to the start of the testosterone injections he told me he usually had fasting sugar levels in the 150 to 180 range. More recently he reported that they have almost all been between 70 and 90.

Not only has Sam's libido returned to a healthy level, but he feels much more energetic, "… jumping out of bed ready to go," as he put it.

For those familiar with the terms and like to know numbers, Sam's HgbA1C (glycohemoglobin) went from 9.2 before the testosterone injections to 8 at his last checkup with no change in his diabetic therapy.

We are going to maintain Sam on the same dosages of his diabetic medications and monitor his HgbA1C every couple of months.

To conclude this section on diabetes I have a couple of testosterone—type II diabetes conjectures:

> Does testosterone deficiency play a predisposing role in developing abdominal obesity?

> Could testosterone deficiency be an integral part of the Metabolic Syndrome? (The Metabolic Syndrome is a term coined within the past couple of decades to describe patients with the commonly associated quartet of abdominal obesity, high blood pressure, insulin resistance [type II diabetes], and lipid abnormalities [abnormal cholesterol and triglycerides]. Coronary artery disease is so common in this group of people that many researchers believe they all should be assumed to have it.)

(Quite recently a medical journal article was brought to my attention which cites studies that have linked testosterone deficiency to type II diabetes and the Metabolic Syndrome. The patients studied in this article were men put into a state of severe testosterone deficiency as part of their treatment for prostate cancer. The full problem of testosterone deficiency and its multiple health ramifications is many thousands of times more common.)

GYNECOMASTIA

Gynecomastia is the growth of breast tissue in the male. It is mentioned in the official FDA warnings concerning testosterone therapy. Gynecomastia is actually a fairly common phenomenon among boys during early puberty. It likely results from breast tissue being stimulated by the initial surge of sexual hormone secretion, mainly testosterone. The breast tissue then shrinks away and essentially disappears as testosterone levels continue to rise. In view of this phenomenon, I would think that any adult male on testosterone therapy who develops gynecomastia is either early in his course of treatment, or is probably getting too small a dose.

I have only recently come to the opinion that gynecomastia may be more common in adult males than any of us realize. The more I check for it, the more of it I find. It might well be the case that many or most men who look like they have breasts, *do* have breasts.

Quite the contrary to the warning about gynecomastia, the patients I have seen with gynecomastia have all had low testosterone levels, and treatment with testosterone has either greatly lessened their breast tissue or made it disappear completely.

Within the past half-year I had a fifty-nine year old male patient with what turned out to be a very feminine problem. I've known him for years, but it never really occurred to me that what looked like breasts on his chest actually were breasts. He came to see me because he had developed a painful lump in his chest. Upon examining him not only did the lump feel like a breast cyst, but the rest of the *fat* on his chest had the feel of breast tissue. He disclosed that he had had essentially no libido for many years.

A mammogram revealed the lump to be consistent with cystic mastitis, an inflamed breast cyst. We also found that he had a very low serum testosterone level. Treatment with testosterone completely eliminated the cyst and, so far, has done away with about two thirds of his breast tissue. How much breast tissue will ultimately disappear remains to be seen. He has also become sexually active with his wife again.

I have another male patient, also fifty-nine years old, who many months ago complained of an ill defined sense of swelling over the right side of his chest extending into his armpit. Visually, the right side of his chest was slightly more prominent. To the touch, his chest felt like it was full of breast tissue. This man also had a low testosterone level and admitted to a marked decline in his interest in sex during the past few years. His story proved to be the same. His serum testosterone level was low, and treatment eliminated his chest swelling and recharged his sex life.

GYNECOLOGICAL: FIBROIDS, MENSTRUAL PERIODS, AND PREGNANCY

Many women have told me that fibroids that they once could feel in their lower abdomen seemed to disappear after several testosterone injections. Many women have also told me that testosterone therapy seemed to lessen their excessive menstrual bleeding. These reports were very interesting, even intriguing, but vague. Two women, however, were able to document their gynecologic effects from testosterone with the help of their gynecologists.

Rosemarie L., a fifty-two year old woman, has been on testosterone replacement therapy for a little over two years. She had always been a very libidinous woman, very sexually active, making love with her husband a major part of her life. She began to lose her physical desire when she was about forty-six, and by forty-nine felt that she was sexually essentially dead. She became depressed, fatigued, and, understandably, some marital problems appeared.

We had many discussions about testosterone, its potential benefits and side effects. She was hesitant and fearful, but her libido showed no signs of revival, and her husband was very frustrated. After about a year of talking and thinking she agreed to try a few testosterone injections.

Rosemarie's sex life changed so drastically after the second injection that the next time she saw me she actually blushed. She came over to me, bent down to whisper in my ear, and with a girlish giggle said, "It's like I'm twenty again."

The normalization of their love life is wonderful, and has continued, but it isn't the point of this story.

Prior to the start of her testosterone treatment Rosemarie was being followed by her gynecologist for an 8 cm. (approx. 3 in.) uterine fibroid, and very heavy menstrual bleeding. During the ensuing two years not only did her excessive bleeding gradually diminished, but her gynecologist told her that the fibroid was getting smaller. For the past eight to twelve months Rosemarie has had normal menstrual periods, ("... like when I was a young woman."), and recently, at her last visit to her gynecologist, was told that her fibroid couldn't be felt.

Evelyn I. is a fifty-three year old mentioned earlier in this chapter. In May of 2005 a pelvic sonogram revealed that she had a small right ovarian cyst.

In March of 2006, within weeks of starting testosterone replacement therapy, another pelvic sonogram was reported as showing an irregular endometrium (internal lining of the uterus), and a mass in the lower portion of her uterus. It was believed to be a fibroid but her gynecologist recommended a procedure to look into her uterus to evaluate the mass. Evelyn declined to have the procedure done.

In October of 2006, after being on testosterone injections for eight months, another pelvic sonogram was reported as being completely normal.

A lessening of menstrual cramping appears to be yet another unexpected effect of testosterone. A few women have reported this phenomenon to me.

One is Cindy E. whose full story is presented in the next chapter. She has suffered with menstrual cramping all her adult life. The problem used to be quite severe, sometimes incapacitating. Since Cindy began getting testosterone she has reported that during many periods she has almost no cramping at all. During many others she only has mild to moderate cramping. On infrequent occasions her cramps have approached the level of her pre-testosterone problem. We are trying to determine if the timing of the testosterone shot is playing any role in the severity of her cramping.

Another patient with a story about menstrual cramping is Linda R. She's a forty-six year old woman who began taking testosterone injections for a failing libido about ten months ago. Since she was acquainted with other women who were receiving testosterone replacement therapy from me she expected to experience a return to the satisfying sexuality she had known years earlier. That was exactly what happened, probably to an even greater degree than she had anticipated. What she had not expected, however, was a major lessening of her menstrual cramps. Linda had dealt with intense cramping, nausea, and vomiting with her menstrual periods for as long as she could remember. Simultaneous with the re-blossoming of her libido came a marked improvement in her menstrual symptoms, so much so that she stated that more than half her pain had disappeared, and the nausea and vomiting were gone completely. Furthermore, Linda informed me that many other women getting testosterone injections were experiencing the same improvement in their menstrual symptoms.

A speculation about a possible role testosterone could possibly play in fertility and pregnancy appears after the case history of Terri H. in Chapter Six.

FIBROMYALGIA AND THE RESTLESS LEG SYNDROME

I've had far too many women patients tell me about significant improvement in their fibromyalgia type muscle pains for me to not speculate that testosterone replacement may help that condition. The case report on Sharon T. in Chapter Six is a prime example.

By its two names, fibromyalgia and fibromyositis, we know that the problem is pain caused by inflamed muscle tissue. There are a few interesting possible connections between this condition and testosterone. Testosterone deficiency problems are much worse in women, and fibromyalgia seems to occur almost exclusively in women. We know that testosterone strengthens muscle cells—it must be making them healthier. The likelihood that testosterone has some positive effect on muscle cell membranes is evidenced by its beneficial effect on type II diabetes. If the pain and inflammation of fibromyalgia is caused by some of the internal contents of the muscle cells leaking out through their membranes, for whatever reason, we have a perfect scenario to understand why testosterone may help. It would be interesting to do a study on the testosterone levels of fibromyalgia sufferers.

The Restless Leg Syndrome is a condition that causes people to suffer from an uncontrollable urge to keep moving their legs when sitting or especially when lying down and trying to sleep. I have never had the sense that this Restless Leg Syndrome is a neurological problem as seems to be the current theory of the medical community. I think more likely it is a very mild form of fibromyalgia, the restlessness coming from trying to find a position to ease a barely discernible discomfort. Here too, therefore, I wonder if there is any connection with testosterone deficiency.

I recently had reason to review the records of a patient I had been seeing for many years. With some surprise I realized that he was the second worst case of testosterone deficiency I've seen, the worst being John C. Al D. is a clarion example of many of the issues I've raised in this book. I've chosen to place his story here because of all his many problems, muscle weakness and pain were the most pronounced.

Al was an active, athletic, thirty-three year old when he first became my patient in 1997. At that time, and during the next seven to eight years, Al had constant complaints of severe fatigue, muscle weakness, and muscular pain. One on occasion he described how difficult it was to hold his infant child in his arms. In 2000 he complained of recurrent bouts of facial flushing. (I was too dumb at the time to realize that the man was going through menopause.) A year after that he complained of a failing libido.

Al also had other chronic complaints. He suffered from ongoing stress, and repeatedly complained of anxiety, the latter so severe at times that it bordered on panic attacks. He was also chronically severely depressed.

During these years Al saw three neurologists, a psychiatrist, and at least two rheumatologists in our search for the cause of his muscle and other problems. No one had a diagnosis for him.

Of all the tests done by all these doctors and myself during all these years, there were three that were noteworthy.

> In April 2002 a rheumatology consultant included a free testosterone level among his large battery of blood tests. The value came back within the laboratory's normal range, but at a level that I now would consider to be insufficient.

> A few months after that Al underwent a muscle biopsy. The pathology report stated that his muscle tissue was minimally abnormal and most consistent with a myopathy (muscle disease).

> CPK is an enzyme made by muscle cells that normally finds its way into the blood in small amounts. Any sort of an injury to muscle tissue raises the blood level of this enzyme. High levels are found during heart attacks, for example, and after muscle trauma. The normal level at a laboratory I use is 0 to 200. Between the end of

2002 and the end of 2004 I did this test on Al twelve times. Not one result was normal. The values ranged from 251 to 557, the average being 348.

After finding an extremely low level of serum testosterone in November of 2004, Al agreed to a trial of replacement therapy. He reported that each injection gave him a strength boost and an ebbing of his muscle pain. From that point on my notes no longer include any complaints of anxiety or depression.

After three injections Al decided to stop because of his fear of prostate cancer. He rapidly relapsed, conceding after only a few months that the strength he had regained from the three doses of testosterone had disappeared.

Al resumed testosterone treatment in April 2006 and again reported a lessening of his muscle pain and an increase in strength after each injection. His libido has improved, he suffers from much less depression, and reports having had no anxiety attacks at all. *His recent CPK done after a long interval was 120.*

There can be no doubt that Al D. had suffered from severe hypogonadism for years. His testosterone deficiency had not only resulted in a whole host of symptoms, but also repeatedly abnormal muscle blood tests and an abnormal muscle biopsy. Despite the severity of his disease, and repeated medical evaluations, he went undiagnosed by at least a half-dozen physicians, including myself, for about seven years.

There are innumerable men and women currently suffering from various consequences of testosterone deficiency. Unlike Al they will remain undiagnosed, likely for their entire lives, unless the private and public medical establishments take a fresh, unbiased, and candid look at all aspects of this disease.

6

Testosterone and Sexual Health

The medical community is guilty of two major failures in regard to sexual health. The first is their failure to find out about it. The second is their failure to do anything about it.

As I briefly alluded to earlier, based only upon my experience in my office there seems to be a general disinclination by primary care physicians and gynecologists to probe into the sex lives of their patients. I use the term, probe, because with most men and women there is initially a reluctance to talk about their libido, their desires, their orgasms or lack of them, and a little encouragement is needed for them to open up. I would emphasize the word, "little". Women, after they've become comfortable with talking about sex, have frequently commented to me, with some annoyance, that their gynecologists never asked them about their sex lives. Men have also often told me that their former physicians never asked them about sex. I understand the reluctance of these doctors to get involved in conversations about sex. It is common to have unfounded complaints filed against doctors, and teachers also, for that matter. I've had fictitious complaints filed against me on a few occasions, although none of a sexual nature. Fortunately, the complaints were all so patently false that it required very little effort to reveal how nonsensical they were.

In the matter of sexual health, however, I also was guilty of neglect. I spent decades avoiding the subject with my patients, but by doing so I partially failed as a physician.

It is an inescapable fact of life and living that doing something about problems with sexual health will most of the time mean replacing testosterone. Many physicians and nurses, probably even most, shy away from testosterone as if the hormone was a cousin to heroin. It's understandable that they'd be very leery considering all the less than favorable media publicity and government policy.

Some of my colleagues are even of the opinion that testosterone may cause prostate cancer. I don't believe that it does. Although no one can say at this point in time that the possibility doesn't exist, injectable testosterone has been around for a very long time, and, as we've seen, the highest official powers that be, those whose job it is to be extremely wary, can't even go to the point of calling the alleged testosterone—prostate cancer connection a possibility, or even a supposition. They can only call it a, "concept". There is much more on the subject of testosterone and prostate cancer in Chapter Eight.

In regard to sex, testosterone has taken on something of a tawdry aura, almost as if it was a sleazy, illicit, drug being used to stimulate some crude, lascivious, sexual high. The reality is that it is a very important hormone being used to treat <u>one</u> of probably several symptoms arising from a disease, the disease being an acquired hormone deficiency.

It would be a very similar situation if thyroid hormone was widely looked upon as being in the same league as the stimulants cocaine and methamphetamine because it relieved the fatigue and sluggishness of hypothyroidism. Incidentally, hypothyroidism also can cause loss of libido. With this disease also, therefore, the reawakening of dormant sexual desire by thyroid hormone replacement could be viewed the same way testosterone seems to be viewed, as an almost illegal stimulant only being administered to enhance sexual pleasure.

This widespread mind-set can have unhappy results. I have a woman patient in her fifties who for a couple of years declined my suggestions that she try testosterone replacement for her chronic fatigue and disinterest in sex. When she finally did take a few injections, she ultimately came to, "… feel healthy physically, sexually, and mentally," as she put it. When she went away for this past summer I gave her a prescription so she would have her own bottle of testosterone with her. Despite having her own testosterone, and my prescription with directions, five physicians and two nurses refused to give her an injection. When she returned to my office after two months without testosterone she was tired, depressed, and had again lost her interest in sex. She was highly incensed and angry, and rightly so, because the reality was that these medical professionals had refused to treat her disease. She had to suffer unnecessarily, but she returned to her "normal" pre-menopausal, pre-hormone deficient, self after a couple of weeks.

Sex, of course, has had one of the two best known and most advertised identifications with testosterone. The other has been the illegal and harmful use by body builders and athletes, the former to bulk up their muscles, the latter to enhance their performance. This limited popular association of testosterone with just these two aspects of medicine shouldn't be surprising for three reasons.

- Superior athletic performance leads to big, big, bucks.

- Sex is one of the primary and most popular instincts of life.

- Research into other consequences of testosterone deficiency doesn't seem to have had much medical interest.

I'll say no more about the athletic use of testosterone except this: *To me the permissive attitude of the governing authorities of professional sports, as evidenced by their blatant, decades long, foot-dragging, approach to the problem, has been incomprehensible and deplorable.*

Testosterone is one of the primary hormones of reproduction, vital to species survival. I'm not knowledgeable enough to comment on the physiologic role of testosterone in pregnancy, but I can say that without testosterone no one would be interested in sexual intercourse, and there wouldn't be any pregnancies. This is certainly not a situation unique to humans. The animals we know of in our everyday lives have zero interest in reproductive activity until their testosterone starts to flow. One only has to watch films of rams, when ewe's are in season, trying to break each others skulls, or stallions trying to kick each other, or bull walruses trying to gash each other to death, to know how powerful the effects of testosterone can be.

Note that in the above examples all the animals I mentioned are male. This also holds true in our society. The reflexive sexual association with testosterone is with the male libido and with male sexual aggressiveness. In men testosterone stimulates sex gland activity, and it is probable that these glands, distended with the components of semen, are interpreted by the brain as the desire/need for sex. This is the way the body usually works. If it needs water, it dries the mouth to make us want to drink. If the bladder or rectum is full, the muscles contract to make us want to empty ourselves. If the body senses nutrition needs, signals are sent to the brain which are interpreted as hunger. Men have no problem understanding their sexuality. They feel the need and want to satisfy it. Since they're basically reacting to one hormone there is little to be confused about.

It takes two to tango, however, as the saying goes. What is it that makes a mare or an ewe want to hold for her partner's affections? It's likely the same thing that leads a human female to want to mate—testosterone.

Two aspects of sexuality need to be clarified before proceeding. The first is that in both sexes there is a lot more to sexual desire and fervor than hormones. The human intellect with its emotions, perceptions, personal preferences, as well as the vagaries of life, are all in the mix. The hormone testosterone, however, provides the basic stimulation, the primal urge, that everything else works upon, modifying and shaping it.

The second is that in men, getting and maintaining an erection is a very different process than having a libido. The libido, however, is the sexual foundation necessary for men to even want an erection.

I've found that many women know very little about their sexuality. It is more complicated and confusing than with the other gender since women are reacting reproductively to both female and male hormones. Many women are surprised by what they learn from a short lecture on the sexual workings of the female body.

During pre-menopausal adult life the ovaries are secreting many hormones. Estrogen, progesterone, and others are responsible for ovulation (the production of eggs) and the preparation of the uterus for pregnancy. The lack of a pregnancy results in a menstrual period and the process starts all over. While these female hormones allow for conception and pregnancy, they have relatively little to do with having sex, or rather with the desire to have sex.

The ovaries also secrete a significant amount of testosterone, and this testosterone stimulates clitoral size, tone, and sensitivity. The clitoris is actually a miniature penis, and like the penis can become engorged with blood. It is the stimulation of the clitoris by testosterone and its subsequent engorgement, that the female brain interprets as a desire for sex—a need to have an orgasm. A somewhat similar situation exists in men. A distended, rigid, penis is much more sensitive than a flaccid one. Female hormones, while necessary for ovulation and pregnancy, don't seem to have any sexually stimulating effect.

At menopause, when the ovaries start to deteriorate as secreting glands, the levels of all the hormones it produces begin to fall. The lower levels of the female hormones bring on the loss of menstrual periods. Sexually, the lower levels of testosterone result in shrinking of the clitoris, loss of libido, loss of orgasmic ability, vaginal dryness, and sexual discomfort. It may well be, as the FDA indirectly suggests by its approved indications for methyltestosterone, that it is the lowering levels of all the hormones that brings on the discomfort of menopausal flushing.

There is, however, a lot more to the testosterone deficiency story in the female of our species than just the effects of menopause in the middle-aged. One of my many testosterone surprises has been finding what seems to be a fairly high incidence of sexual dysfunction due to testosterone deficiency among young women. Extrapolating from my very limited patient population, there are probably an extraordinary number who have minimal or absent sexual desire, who have infrequent orgasms or great difficulty reaching orgasm, or who have never even had an orgasm at all. I believe that some, or much, of this is due to physiologic testosterone deficiency.

Not much consideration of our society's willful blindness to the issues of sex and sexuality is needed to see that the issue is mind-boggling. We saw in Chapter Four that the Federal Drug Administration goes through bizarre machinations, defying simple logic, in order to avoid those subjects. In Chapter Three we saw that the laboratories simply will not recognize the existence of a condition of female testosterone deficiency. In this Chapter we learned of the collaboration of the medical establishment. They don't ask, they don't see, they don't want to even hear the word, "testosterone".

This mind-set is so incredibly deep-rooted that even those suffering from the effects of testosterone deficiency don't want to know about it. There haven't been many times during over forty years of asking patients, "How do you feel?" that I heard the reply, "Fine, but I lost my desire for sex."

Most people aren't trying to hide their loss of libido, they're simply refusing to recognize it. The lost lusts of youth are not in the active memory of a forty-five or fifty-five year old. If questioned about their love life their answers are, "We don't really have the time." "The kids are in the house." "We work all day." "Life is so busy." "We're tired." There is no end to their self-deceiving excuses for the loss of their sexuality. At no point do these people choose to recall if work, or a hectic schedule, or fatigue, or other people in the house, stopped them from doing it when they were twenty-two.

The first step in rekindling some of the fires of youth from the embers of middle age is the admission of having cooled off. In many cases, however, those fires had never even been lit in the first place.

SEXUAL HEALTH CASE REPORTS—THE MORE MATURE SET

The success rate of injected testosterone in stimulating a failed libido is exceedingly high. Indeed, the failures I have encountered can almost be counted on the fingers of one hand. They are discussed in Chapter Seven.

Some words of warning are advisable before the reader proceeds through this section. Many, even most, people, especially women, experience a rush during the early stages of testosterone replacement. They enjoy a sense of almost super-well-being. They feel extraordinarily charged up mentally, physically, and sexually. It's really a sign of just how profoundly deprived of testosterone their bodies have been. In a real sense they're going through the excitement of puberty all over again. One man in his early forties is even going through a voice change. His serum testosterone level was extremely low, so low that in all probability he never fully completed his sexual maturation as a teen. After we discussed what was likely happening with him, his concern over his slight hoarseness and voice cracking changed to an anticipation of having a deeper, nicer, voice.

Just as the intense heat of puberty doesn't last forever, neither does this initial rush from testosterone replacement. Eventually, some months after the start of therapy, I'll usually hear something to the effect that the last shot didn't seem to work as well. Often the patient wants a larger dose. Much of the time, however, increasing the amount of testosterone isn't the answer. What is needed is an acceptance of how the body works, an acceptance of feeling thirty instead of eighteen. Many patients, having lost the physical and sexual high of that first surge of hormone replacement, slip into the opinion that the testosterone really isn't working anymore so why bother with the shots? They've forgotten how they felt before the first injection. That recollection is abundantly revived when they return to being hormonally deprived again. Almost all of these patients come back to renew their therapy. If anybody really wanted to re-experience the initial high of testosterone replacement, they'd have to first stop taking the hormone completely for a year or two in order to re-adapt themselves to being testosterone deficient. It's hardly worth it.

Following are some case histories of real people, only the names have been changed. Their stories are representative of the many, many, dozens of patients I have treated over the years.

When I asked Ronald C., a gentleman in his late fifties, about his sex life a couple of years ago, he laughingly related that he had little to none, that he had, "long had no need", as he put it. He admitted that he would certainly like to have a sex life again, but his wife had no interest so why should he bother? When I suggested that I discuss it with her he burst out laughing. He couldn't imagine that she would have any interest in getting, "sex shots", as he put it.

Mrs. C. is also my patient, a very prim and proper lady indeed, but I did raise the subject with her during the course of her next visit and to my surprise she enthusiastically agreed to try the testosterone injections, right there and then.

Within months these two had an active sex life again, so much so that the gentleman told me his wife would sometimes wake him up in the middle of the night to have relations. Mrs. C. ultimately stopped the injections because of facial hair growth, one of many women who seem to panic at the first sign of hair and don't have the patience to see what lowering the dose of testosterone will accomplish. There is much more on this subject later. Ronald, however, still comes in regularly for his shots and tells me that they are still sexually active.

Sharon T. is a professional woman in her early fifties. She was referred to me by a sex therapist who is familiar with my experience with testosterone. Sharon had been ambivalent about sex her entire life. Although she began to have sexual relations during her late teens, she had never had a significant libido and never had spontaneous sexual thoughts. She stated that she did have an occasional weak orgasm, but only engaged in sex to satisfy her husband. Her sex life had come to a complete end ten years before her visit to me, after she had both of her ovaries removed.

Like almost all of my patients Sharon was very skeptical that testosterone would have an effect on her sexual desires, or rather the lack of them, but she was willing to try.

The turnabout in this woman was dramatic, to say the least. After two doses of testosterone she became highly sexually stimulated, began enjoying intense orgasms, and began fantasizing about sex for the first time in her life. "I'm almost always thinking about it," she said in amazement

The testosterone seems to have also done something else to Sharon. She had suffered from severe muscle pain for many years, and those pains, she told me, had almost disappeared.

Sharon had enough noticeable effect of her lifelong testosterone deficiency, namely her absent libido, and enough education, to have realized for most of her life that something was probably wrong with her. Often, when the deficiency is only mild to moderate, there is no realization of the problem at all, as the next case demonstrates.

Doug Y. is a man in his fifties who has been a patient of mine for many years. He has some medical problems and comes to see me for a checkup about every three months. As has become my habit during recent years I questioned him about his libido during almost every visit. He always replied very positively and emphatically that his libido and sex life were just fine. He had no problems.

More recently, however, his wife indicated, quite clearly and explicitly, that as far as she was concerned such was not the case. They were having relations once or twice a month, or less.

When I questioned Doug about the frequency of his marital relations he agreed with his wife. I advised him that most sexually active people had sex a little more often than once a month, and that I was going to check his testosterone level.

Doug's free testosterone level came back in the range I consider to be deficient. He was surprised by this. He still didn't believe that there was anything wrong with him. I suggested he might try a few injections of testosterone to see if it made any difference. Doug was extremely doubtful that he needed hormone replacement therapy, (he really thought the whole business was nonsense), but he agreed to try it.

I ask all my patients about what effects they're having from the testosterone at every visit. In Doug's case he advised me after about the third shot, in a not very convincing way, that they were working. I heard this same unenthusiastic response at every visit for a couple of months. It sounded like he was just telling me what he thought I wanted to hear. Finally, I called him on it. I'm dialoguing this because he really surprised me.

I was sitting on the stool in the examining room finishing writing my notes while Doug was standing a few feet away buttoning his shirt. "Doug," I said with just a hint of exasperation, "Could you please give me a little more detail about what you're experiencing?"

Doug took a couple of steps to be right in front of me. He bent down to look me straight in the eyes, our faces less than two feet apart, and said: "I've never been so sexually stimulated in my entire life. I've never had orgasms like this, even as a young man. It's like night and day. Every man should get these shots."

Well, I got my answer. Doug had honestly believed that he had always had a normal libido, a normal sex life, but his dramatic response to testosterone therapy is indicative of him having had a lifelong, mild to moderate, deficiency. This is undoubtedly a very common condition in both sexes.

Ralph I. is a youthful appearing gentleman only in his very early fifties. During his initial visit to my office he admitted that he hadn't had much of a sex life for quite a while. He wanted one. His testosterone level, not surprisingly, came back low.

Ralph was very hesitant to try testosterone replacement therapy, and not a little skeptical about having any benefit. Eventually he decided to give it a shot. After only two modest doses he was absolutely delighted that he had suddenly gotten well past a weight lifting plateau at the gym, a goal that had eluded him for a long time. He was also more than a little pleased that his morning erections had reappeared after many years of absence, and that his intimate relations with his wife had gone from, "Once a year to once a week."

At his next visit Ralph's comments were: "I'm taking off at the gym. I put on four pounds." "Now we're getting together (with his wife) two or three times a week. Whenever we have the time. It's like I'm eighteen again."

It seems likely that Ralph is a bit over-stimulated, a very uncommon effect in men. We've reduced his dose of testosterone.

Fay L. is a fifty-seven year old woman who has had sexual problems her entire life. While not subjected to intercourse, she was the victim of repeated physical sexual abuse as a child. Rather than ever trying to analyze her sex problem, Fay always kept pushing it to the back of her mind. Probably she was hesitant to dredge up unpleasant memories. As a result she had never defined it for herself. All she knew was that she had major difficulty having orgasms as a younger woman, and those she did have were weak. The passage of time had made matters worse. During the past five to ten years she'd had no orgasms at all. After some brief hesitation she decided that it might not be a bad idea to probe her psyche. It turned out that for Fay self-analysis while discussing her emotions with someone else was much easier than doing it alone.

It didn't take very long for Fay to realize that she had spent her entire adult life being greatly influenced by an inhibition to let go, to let an orgasm happen. She had even been this way while masturbating. She also was able to recall that even when she was younger and having one of her infrequent orgasms, she seemed to willfully limit its intensity.

The effect of testosterone injections on Fay was remarkable. She had a major surge in her libido, became very well lubricated, but most important of all, at least in regard to her sexual relations with the man in her life, her inhibitions completely disappeared. "I was able to get into it and let go."

The onset of routine intense orgasms had a major effect to strengthen her current relationship.

While the correction of testosterone deficiency has many profound beneficial effects on the physical and mental health of older people, (We'll arbitrarily define that as over seventy.), their age needn't and shouldn't preclude using the hormone for sexual reasons.

Celia R. was mentioned in the section on vaginitis. To re-introduce her, she is in her seventies, a very attractive, young at heart, woman. Unhappy with the effects of aging, with the loss of her love life and her worsening fatigue, she wanted to know if she could obtain the same benefit from testosterone that her peri-menopausal daughter was enjoying. While her sexuality was the primary reason we started Celia on testosterone, chronic fatigue was another major consideration.

Celia's companion of many, many, years is Harry S. He was in his mid-seventies at the time. This is the same gentleman who appeared to relapse and is discussed in the section on adult onset diabetes. Not only had Harry had absolutely no libido for many years, but during the year prior to beginning the testosterone injections he had also begun vocalizing complaints of morning fatigue and occasional shortness of breath when walking.

Neither Celia nor Harry consider themselves to be old. They're both young in heart and mind, and not at all bad in body. Glandular failure had brought an end to an important part of their relationship, and both wanted to see if it could be regained.

When the testosterone kicked in Celia began wanting, and having, sexual relations about twice a week, easily having orgasms. Her whole attitude changed. She was no longer depressed. She felt younger and much more energetic. There's always a smile on her face now. She was also very happy that Harry was so much less grouchy!

Celia's sex life was temporarily interrupted by Harry's "relapse", but she continued to feel physically and mentally better. Now that his relapse is over they're again having frequent relations, and the smile on her face is even broader. In regard to the most current Harry, "He's like a different person. What a blessing."

Obviously, Harry had also regained his libido and his sex life after a few injections of testosterone. He also noticed a significant increase in his strength when at the gym, found that he could walk much longer distances, completely lost his shortness of breath, and felt much less grumpy. (This is another instance of testosterone replacement eliminating shortness of breath, the only logical reason being an increase in heart muscle strength.)

Harry's apparent relapse turned out to be inadvertently over treated diabetes, as was discussed in that chapter. After the discontinuance of the diabetes pill Harry became even more active. He's doing a lot of walking with no fatigue and no shortness of breath, has an abundant libido, and Celia is no longer frustrated.

Cathy M. was a pre-menopausal woman in her early fifties when I first asked her about her sex life a few years ago. She was obviously uncomfortable with the question, much more so than most women are, but after a struggle with some apparent inner turmoil she managed to indicate that she didn't have much of a physical relationship. Moments later, after admitting that she had never had an orgasm, she began crying.

I felt terrible, but pursued what was behind this unexpected emotional outburst. It took some prying. She didn't want to talk. I told her that whatever it was that was going on, talking about it could only make it better. Her face cracked into a bit of a smile when I reassured her that no matter what she told me I wouldn't call the police. The smile apparently breached some psychological barrier and she finally revealed that for years as a young girl she had been sexually abused by a relative. I was the first and only person she had ever told about it.

I advised her that she really needed to see a therapist to work out her years of repression.

At the moment, however, Cathy was very interested to learn about testosterone and its sexual effects on women. We discussed it at length. She wanted to be treated to see if she could have a normal sex life, and we decided to give it a try.

As it turned out, only one injection of testosterone gave Cathy the ability to have orgasms, and for several years now she has remained orgasmic without any further injections. Whether it was the testosterone that improved her sex life, or the catharsis of finally telling someone what had happened to her as a child, or both, I don't know. It does prove, however, the major disservice physicians provide their patients when they do not question them about their sex lives.

I think a satisfying sex life is important even for those without a partner. Cindy E. is in her early forties and not involved with a man. She found my questioning her about her sex life to be very embarrassing. Her initial response was that she didn't have a boyfriend. She expected that to be the end of the subject. She really colored when I pursued the topic and asked her about masturbation. I continued talking in order to give her a chance to collect herself, expounding on the facts that having orgasms is very good for mental and physical health, and that it was my opinion that everybody is entitled to as satisfying a sex life as they can get, even if they're single. Very quickly we were having a conversation about her solo sex life, almost as if we were talking about a cold or a headache—almost.

It turned out that for her entire adult life her sexuality had been more a source of frustration to her than enjoyment. It was very difficult for her to have an orgasm, and when she did climax it was weak. She had never been truly sexually satisfied. Her testosterone level came back low by my standards, and she readily agreed to try replacement therapy.

Cindy's response to the hormone was substantial. She developed a much more active libido, and easily had much more intense orgasms. I could see in her face that she was a happier, less depressed, more content, person. There's more. As reported in Chapter Five, during most of her menstrual periods she has noticed a marked lessening of her chronic severe cramping.

Some people find it very difficult to accept the fact that, to a major degree, we feel the way our hormones mandate us to feel. I have one woman patient in her late forties, well educated, who was very distressed that she had lost essentially all her libido. We discussed testosterone replacement a few times but she was very hesitant to try it. This is a very common and understandable reaction, even a desirable one. People should carefully consider what they do.

This woman, however, also had a strong disbelief that her libido could be affected by testosterone injections. It was almost as if she was affronted by the concept that her desires and emotions were nothing more than a chemical reaction dependent upon the quantity of a certain hormone in her blood. There was one reality she knew well, however, nothing else existed that could possibly stimulate her love life. She decided she might as well try testosterone.

This woman had terrific effects from modest doses of the hormone, so much so that she was embarrassed about it. Yet despite my lecturing that the sexual effect would probably disappear if she stopped the treatment, she repeatedly stops coming for the shots every time they begin to work well. When she does reappear in my office I can see her frustration on her face. She's disappointed that she relapsed. She's not happy with the fact that hormones have such control over her body and her feelings. She feels that she should be libidinous without having to take shots. How utterly unrealistic.

SEXUAL HEALTH CASE REPORTS—THE YOUNGER SET

Lorraine L. was in her late twenties several years ago when she confided unhappily that she had never had an orgasm in her life. (You can learn a lot about a patient when you ask.) She was a single girl, had a boyfriend, and had been sexually active since she was a teenager. On occasion she believed that she had come close to having an orgasm, but it had never triggered. From the tone of our discussion it was obvious that the problem had been a source of frustration to her for a long time.

Lorraine's free testosterone level came back low. We discussed the situation several times during the next many months. I told her that I thought it was possible that the low level of the hormone was preventing her from having an orgasm. Her clitoris simply might not be sensitive enough. I believed that some tesosterone would increase her sensitivity but I didn't know if that would actually accomplished what she wanted. I also told her that I thought sexual fulfillment was important to a person's physical and mental health, and that mutual sexual satisfaction would have a positive effect on her relationship.

Lorraine was understandably hesitant to try the shots but ultimately, understanding the possible consequences should she become pregnant, and that she had to remain on oral contraceptives, agreed to try the hormone.

I don't recall if it was after her first or second injection that I walked into the examination room, and she looked up at me and dryly stated, "So that's what sex is all about."

Apparently, her journey into full sexual enjoyment had come about suddenly, easily, and to her, surprisingly. "It just ... happened." Lorraine also noted an easing of her life. She was less anxious, less depressed, more content. She received one or two more small doses of testosterone, continued to easily have orgasms, then discontinued the treatment, but remained orgasmic until she moved away and I lost contact.

Donna G. is another young woman in her twenties. She's married and the mother of a toddler. She was/is having major trouble with her marriage because of her complete disinterest in sex. She frankly admitted this to me—absolutely no desire. Her testosterone level was very low for someone her age. I tried for a couple of years to get her to try testosterone therapy. A year or so ago she finally did agree to have a couple of injections. She very quickly, and happily, developed an active and satisfying libido. Then she stopped coming to the office.

The next time I saw her she admitted that she had again lost all interest in sex and wasn't having relations with her husband. The reason she had stopped, from what I could surmise, was simply because of what she had been told by her friends.

We started all over again. She began taking testosterone injections a second time. The very first shot had a significant stimulating effect on her, but after the second injection she once again stopped coming to the office. I didn't know why. When I asked other members of her family, they shrugged. They apparently didn't understand her either.

When Donna came to the office recently with a sore throat I learned what had happened. It seems the second injection had a very major effect on her libido. She became very desirous and orgasmic. Even after several months she was still feeling some of the effect. Her marital problems, however, run much deeper than their sex life. She simply doesn't care to be with her husband.

I think the above cases point out something very important. When it comes to sex, testosterone deficiency not only results in the inability to want or enjoy sexual relations, it also has profound personal social consequences. One hormone deficient partner can lead to a failed relationship or even divorce. Although it may not matter very much to Donna, some other woman's disinterest in sex might quite possibly lead to her husband leaving her. Why would any young man want to stay with a woman who refuses to have a love life with him?

From the above you can see that I don't believe testosterone deficiency in the young is limited to women. There are undoubtedly many, many, relatively young men out there who have limited, or no, interest in sex. With this gender the long-term consequences of testosterone deficiency may be even more devastating than a failed relationship. There's more on the subject testosterone deficiency in young males in the section on prostate cancer.

I normally don't begin to question patients about their sexuality until they're at least in their mid-twenties. Marlene R. was a rare exception. At twenty she was a blatantly unhappy, distressed, girl. Her life seemed to revolve around her multiple ongoing complaints of stress, anxiety, depression, chronic fatigue, all symptoms commonly associated with testosterone deficiency. I had no way of knowing at what age symptoms of testosterone deficiency can begin to manifest themselves, but Lorraine L. had apparently begun to become symptomatic in her teens.

Marlene was understandably initially very embarrassed to talk about her sexuality. People who have no sex problems simply reply in the negative when I first broach the subject, and that's the end of it. Marlene didn't do that.

I've found that in the ticklish situation of embarrassment the best policy is to immediately stop talking about sex and openly air and discuss the embarrassment itself. The patient can then choose to return to the subject of sex or not. It is rare that young women with a sex problem do not want to talk about it, and Marlene wasn't rare.

We were able to break the ice by agreeing that if there was anything about her love life that could possibly lend itself to discussion, then very obviously all was not well. That opened the floodgates.

It turned out that she had been sexually active for several years, sometimes with a male partner and often by herself, but she wasn't sure if she had ever had an orgasm. It bothered her. (If someone isn't sure if they've ever had an orgasm or not, they haven't, at least not a full one.)

Marlene's testosterone level was below what I consider to be adequate, and after my experience with Lorraine L. and Cathy M., I wondered if just a couple of small doses of testosterone might be enough to activate her orgasm mechanism on a more or less permanent basis. After we discussed the dangers of pregnancy and determined that she had no man in her life at the time, she was very willing to try a couple of testosterone injections.

The first shot had little if any effect. She wasn't sure. After the second injection, however, I didn't see Marlene again for six or seven months. I had assumed that she was one of those rare patients who don't respond to testosterone. I was wrong. It turned out that the second injection had not only made her understand what she had been missing from sex all her young mature life, but had also put her in a much better, happier, less nervous, frame of mind. The effect had lasted many, many months and had only recently begun to fade. Since she is on oral contraceptives and is still not active with a partner, we decided that for the time being one or two small doses a couple of times a year was worth the significant physical and psychological benefit.

While on this subject of young women getting testosterone; patients and colleagues have often voiced their concern about the hormone affecting young women's menstrual cycles or their ovulation. I have seen some minor effects of this nature, but nothing major. Let's take a step back and consider the broader picture. Women's ovaries are producing female and male hormones. People raise concern about the male hormone, testosterone, affecting their menstrual cycle, but no one thinks twice about the millions of these women taking female hormones, estrogens and progesterones, for many years in the form of oral contraceptives for the express purpose of affecting their menstrual cycles and ovulation. There seems to be a hormonal double standard here.

Ellen S. is a mother in her mid-thirties who has complained to me for many years about chronic tiredness and listlessness. Even several years ago, when she was in her very early thirties, she related that she had minimal desire to have sex. The problem may have even pre-dated that.

During a recent visit she confided that now she basically had no sexual desire at all and had no enjoyment from sex. Since Ellen is trying to get pregnant she's not a candidate for testosterone treatment, but we decided to check her serum level anyway so she can consider some future decisions. It is very low. Her serum testosterone level came back as the lowest number the laboratory reports. Anything less simply gets the "<" sign before the number.

There is no doubt but that Ellen S., at the age of thirty, and probably even younger, was symptomatic of testosterone hormone deficiency. It cannot be that this is an uncommon problem among young women if I am seeing so many in my practice. Based upon the responses of many, many, other women, if Ellen was able to be treated with testosterone she would become energized, perhaps more than she has ever been as an adult, have a more positive frame of mind, and begin to enjoy sex, and life, to a much fuller extent.

The case of Terri H. is included only because of a speculative connection between testosterone and pregnancy which is discussed in the paragraph following her story.

Very simply, Terri is in her early forties, has a history of having had a miscarriage many, many, years ago, and now has been trying to get pregnant for over a year without success. She is still menstruating, has female hormonal levels in the middle of their normal ranges, but, by my standards, has a low testosterone level. I haven't questioned her about her libido.

I hope I continue to see these two women. I am very interested to see if they can have a successful pregnancy with their low testosterone levels. During the past several years I've had reason to wonder if there was any connection between fertility problems in women and their testosterone levels. Since I had no plans to write a book about the hormone at the time, those patients who generated that consideration in my mind are long lost from memory. With testosterone apparently having a very significant effect on the uterus by shrinking fibroids, normalizing menstrual bleeding, and lessening menstrual cramping, there is certainly the possibility of some connection between the hormone and the ability of a uterus to hold a successful pregnancy.

Following is a list of what I've seen in the way of sexual effects of testosterone therapy in women.
> Marked increase in libido and ease and strength of orgasms.
> Marked increase in thick mucous vaginal lubrication.
> Marked decrease in any discomfort with intercourse.
> Marked increase in breast erotic sensitivity.

7

Treatment

The only sensible and effective treatment for testosterone deficiency is testosterone replacement. There are three ways to get the hormone into the body, by pills, by topical application on the skin, and by injection. Some vaginal creams contain testosterone but it is applied there for the local effect, not as a means to enter the body. Let me clearly state up front that I have little to no experience with the first two forms of therapy, so my comments that follow are primarily based upon impressions that I have gained over the years.

The natural, unadulterated, hormone, testosterone, is not absorbed very well. The oral form of the hormone is an altered molecule, methyltestosterone. To the best of my knowledge the absorption of even this variety of the hormone is not reliable or predictable, and since it is my understanding that it cannot be measured in the blood, there is no way to know how much of the hormone is actually getting into the body. Furthermore, there is some risk of liver toxicity with this compound. It is therapy totally in the dark, and I do not prescribe it.

There has been much publicity lately about studies done with a testosterone cream or patch. The beneficial effects have been positive, but, as I understand the reports, not nearly to the degree that I have experienced with testosterone injections. I don't know if the transdermal (through the skin) absorption of this form of testosterone is predictable and measurable.

The advantages of depository testosterone injections are that we know *exactly* how much of the hormone is getting into the body, and we can adjust that amount by dosage and timing to any degree. Furthermore, the injections result in <u>cyclic</u> quantities of testosterone in the body. The levels rise rapidly right after an injection then slowly fall off during the following weeks. There are several possible advantages to this.

> In the female it may mimic cyclic secretions of testosterone by the ovaries. The secretions of the other ovarian hormones are cyclic, and it only makes sense for the levels of testosterone to be the highest when an egg is present for fertilization. (Nature is deeply rooted in common sense.)

> In both sexes, when we see a definitive lessening of the sexual effect of the testosterone before the next dose we know that the dose hasn't been excessive.

> In both sexes, a temporary mild deficiency state lasting a few days before the next shot may re-sensitize cell receptors to make the subsequent dose work well, and may also allow for some pituitary stimulation to keep that gland awake. (The taking of any hormone that is regulated by the pituitary gland results in the slowing or shutting down of that pituitary activity. For example, the pituitary hormone TSH [thyroid stimulating hormone] regulates how much thyroid hormone is secreted by the thyroid gland. If thyroid hormone is taken in the form of a pill, the pituitary senses this and slows or stops the production of TSH.)

The dose of intramuscular depository testosterone I've been using for men has been 300 mg to 400 mg, every three to four weeks. The beneficial effects on men are much less apparent than with women, and other than testicular shrinkage (discussed later) there haven't been any untoward side effects.

I had anticipated the possibility of testosterone leading some men to develop a problem with their prostate. The hormone might cause some swelling of that gland that could cause symptoms of urinary obstruction. I've questioned men with mild pre-existing prostate problems very carefully to ascertain if the testosterone was making them any worse, but after many years I've encountered nothing of significance. This not to say that it can't happen to some men, but the potential seems to be very small.

A study on this topic, authored by Dr. Leonard S. Marks from UCLA, appeared in the most recent issue of JAMA, the Journal of the American Medical Association. Dr. Marks has kindly given me permission to quote from his article.

Concern over the safety of testosterone replacement therapy (TRT) in older men prompted the study. The specific object of the study was to determine the effects of TRT on prostate tissue of aging men with low serum testosterone levels. Adverse effects were looked for in many ways, including prostate biopsies. Although the dose of testosterone used in this study was lower than the dose I use in my office, the following are the conclusions of the study.

"These preliminary data suggest that in aging men with late-onset hypogonadism, 6 months of TRT normalizes serum androgen levels but appears to have little effect on prostate tissue androgen levels and cellular functions. Establishment of prostate safety for large populations of older men undergoing longer duration of TRT requires further study."

My experience with testosterone therapy in women has been quite the opposite in all aspects. There seems to be a significant variation in dose requirements, anywhere from 20 mg to 100 mg. Some of that may be due to some women seeking a greater sexual high and exaggerating their need. The therapeutic theme in my office is always to take the smallest amount that will provide a satisfactory effect.

The beneficial effects on women are much more pronounced and dramatic than with men, as are the side effects. The latter is discussed in the Side Effects section in Chapter Eight. The degree of sexual arousal in women is far more striking, as is their feeling of increased energy and well-being. I suspect this is due to the same reason women have so much worse osteoporosis. Most testosterone deficient men still have a substantial amount of the hormone in them, while deficient women may have almost none, or even amounts that are undetectable.

The first dose of testosterone seldom does anything, although an occasional man or woman does report some vague stirrings. In experimenting with the timing of subsequent injections I've found that if it is given less often than every four weeks we approach a situation where every shot is a first dose. An injection given every four weeks can maintain some significant therapeutic response. A dose given every three weeks will build to, and maintain, a good therapeutic response with a few cooling off days during each treatment period. This is the timing I recommend to my patients. The largest dose according to the official prescribing information for men is 400 mg every two weeks.

One more observation about treatment. As was noted in some of the above case reports, it may be that in some people a limited treatment course with testosterone triggers some permanent or semi-permanent change in their chemistry, and they maintain the beneficial effects for some period of time when the injections are discontinued.

TREATMENT FAILURES

I have had some treatment failures, but so few that I can almost count them on one hand.

One such patient was a woman in her seventies who was complaining only about excessive fatigue. Apparently, she has lived with a very intense libido all her life, and with even the smallest dose of testosterone she became so sexually aroused that no matter how much she tried to satisfy herself the arousal remained with her constantly. We discontinued treatment and she returned to normal.

Another woman, seventy-six years old, denied that she had noticed any improvement in her fatigue or anything else even after about five injections of testosterone. We stopped them several months ago. Recently, however, she brought up the subject of the testosterone shots, suggesting that we try them again. She may prove to be another instance of the phenomenon of unnoticed improvement.

Two other failures were men, both suffering from rather severe chronic depressive problems, far beyond your average, every day, type of depression. One of them had an extremely low serum testosterone level, well below even the laboratory's lower limits of normal. Despite a multiple injection trial there was no noticeable effect of testosterone on either one of them. *I do have the strong sense that commonly used antidepressants can block the appreciation of any effects of testosterone replacement.*

DISCONTINUANCE AND RETURN TO THERAPY

As my experience with testosterone replacement therapy has grown I've noticed that quite a few patients, more than I would have expected, who had discontinued testosterone injections for various reasons, eventually returned and asked for the treatment to be resumed. Sometimes patients would tell me at the time of their decision why they were discontinuing the hormone. I learned about others by questioning them during the course of an office visit for some other purpose. Still others explained their reason when they came back to resume treatment.

Most of the patients who stopped their testosterone therapy were women who couldn't tolerate their facial hair growth and closed their minds. I cannot recall one woman who was unable to find a dose of testosterone that provided significant benefit and minimal, or no, hair growth problems. I found no risk to this approach. All new facial hair growth disappeared completely on all of my female patients who stopped taking testosterone. Other patients have stopped the treatment on the advice of friends, or because of what they heard from relatives.

(I have always found it absolutely amazing how many, many, people have friends and relatives whom they regard as being experts in almost every field of medicine. These people attentively listen to, and heed, their friends'/relatives' opinions and advice. What's even more amazing is that if you ask these people if their friend or relative really knows anything at all about the subject at hand, they invariably reply in the negative.)

Some women, like the case reported as a treatment failure, have stopped taking testosterone because they found the sexual stimulation uncomfortable. They had no partner to satisfy their need, were disinclined to masturbate, and preferred to be asexual. Some patients stopped the injections because they didn't like the idea of taking hormone shots forever. They feared the ultimate appearance of some as yet unknown side effect. Finally, some patients stopped coming for shots because they felt that they weren't working—they felt nothing different, no better. Some of these are reported in the discussion of unnoticed improvement in the "Fatigue" section of Chapter Five.

As reported in that section, many of these latter patients who felt that the shots weren't doing anything for them ultimately came to realize, once the effects of the last dose had fully worn off, that there had indeed been a major benefit. Others returned to treatment because the feeling of physical and sexual well-being that they had experienced, and now lacked, overrode other negative considerations. Finally, some women resumed their treatment because someone had come into their life and they wanted to be, and feel, sexually alive.

ETHICS

Some might see my treatment of testosterone deficiency as nothing more than providing people with a hormonal high, a sexual rush, using testosterone as a drug rather than just as a replacement. My counter to that possibility is that I have been giving them about the same amount of testosterone that their own glands used to provide them when they were younger (unless they had been under active all their lives).

I happened across a body-building web site recently. The main article was a discourse on the dosages, potential problems, and alternatives to the parent compound, testosterone. The largest dose men took for the purpose of body building, according to this article, was four grams (4,000 mg) of testosterone per week. I have never even given any man the FDA approved full dose of 400 mg every two weeks, but limit it to a three week interval. These men are taking thirty times (30 X) more testosterone than I give my male patients. They are looking for a different type of response from testosterone than I am. I'm replacing a missing hormone to regain its natural physical and mental effects. They are looking for an unnatural stimulation of their muscle cells for the purpose of making them grow as large as possible

As with drugs and alcohol, when some type of chemical is taken to produce an effect greater than what nature intended, the target tissue or cells tend to become refractory or numb to the effect, and ever increasing doses are required to get the high. I have seen absolutely no instances where increasingly larger doses of testosterone were needed to maintain a therapeutic effect.

8

Side Effects and Prostate Cancer

When considering reported side effects of testosterone keep in mind that in both sexes there are two distinctly different groups of people receiving testosterone therapy. One group is receiving physiologic doses of the hormone which are simply replacing what their own glands are no longer secreting. The other group is taking mega-doses as was mentioned in the previous chapter, as much as thirty times (3,000 %) more than the first group, in order to increase their muscle mass or athletic ability. In some instances the side effect Warnings and Precautions address the difference between these two groups, but for the most part they do not.

SIDE EFFECTS IN WOMEN

All medical treatments, of course, have potential side effects. As has been mentioned many times earlier, in the case of testosterone administration to women the major consideration is the avoidance of the hormone during pregnancy.

By far the major side effect complaint from women is facial hair growth. This is common, at least to some degree. Keep in mind, however, that a good many women have very little in the way of facial hair follicles. In their skin there is almost nothing for the testosterone to stimulate.

The degree of hair growth for those prone to this side effect is entirely dose dependent, and I have always seen it to be completely reversible. Unfortunately, quite a few women who had extremely good responses to the first few injections of testosterone abruptly discontinued them after developing facial hair growth. They seemed to panic at the presence of the facial hair and close their minds. Their reaction was unwarranted. Those who had the patience to see the effects of lowered doses almost all ultimately found the dose that provided them with meaningful physical and sexual benefit and absent or tolerable facial hair growth. In any event, again, I have never had a female patient who didn't completely lose all new facial hair after stopping testosterone no matter how long they took it.

One woman patient in her fifties who has been getting testosterone injections for quite some time was quite opinionated on the matter of hair growth. She seemed almost incensed at what she considered the "silliness" of other women, but was quite flattered when I asked her to repeat her comment because I was going to quote her.

"I don't understand why women are so afraid of facial hair. Most women are going to get facial hair anyway. I think it's a very minor trade-off. There isn't a part of the body that can't be waxed or shaved or lasered or something. Why give up feeling so much better?"

It should also be noted that it is not uncommon for the rate of facial hair growth to lessen over time even if the same dose of testosterone is continued.

As will be seen in Chapter Nine I believe that menopausal women should also be taking female hormones, quite possibly for their entire lives. It could be the case that with the addition of female hormones to testosterone the problem of facial hair growth might be lessened considerably.

The second most common undesirable side effect I have seen in women is sexual over stimulation. Until the right dose is found some women simply become excessively aroused. They're distracted by sexual thoughts all day. It is a problem, but one that is easily and quickly correctable, and also one they laugh about.

The third most common complaint from women is probably weight gain. Early on it was a mystery to me why many women were gaining a bit of weight. There is certainly some appetite stimulation from testosterone, but most of these women were swearing that their eating habits hadn't changed. I've listened to enough weight stories over the past forty years to gauge the truth of what I'm told.

One day a woman, even though she said her waist seemed to have slimmed, was complaining bitterly about her inability to lose the few pounds she had gained. She went to the gym so often, she said, and exercised so hard! A thought struck me. I asked her to lift her dress so I could see her legs. Her muscles were firm, even hard. The woman was exercising so much that while her fat was disappearing, with the testosterone in her she was simply getting stronger, adding new muscle. Muscle cells are full of water, and water is very, very, *heavy*, much heavier than fat. There's also the likelihood that women on testosterone replacement are laying down new bone, they're reversing their osteoporosis, and bone is even heavier than water.

It would be the height of foolishness to forego the beneficial effects of testosterone replacement simply because of some number on a scale, a number that's actually indicating that you are getting stronger and healthier!

There have been occasional other side effects such as acne, voice deepening, and slight personality changes, but these have been very minimal, dependent on the dose used, and reversible.

SIDE EFFECTS IN MEN

The common side effect of testosterone replacement in men is testicular shrinkage. The size of the testes is normally maintained by stimulating hormones coming from the pituitary gland. The response of the testes to these hormones in the matter of testosterone production has become inadequate which is the reason these men have become testosterone deficient. The pituitary gland senses the higher blood testosterone levels coming from the injections and decreases the production of its hormones. This causes the testes to shrink a bit. In my experience it has always been a reversible phenomenon. In the end the choice is between having enough testosterone to have energy, strength, a full libido, and an active sex life, with slightly smaller testes, or insufficient testosterone, weakness and fatigue, little or no libido and sex, and normal sized testes.

Prostate Cancer

The possibility that testosterone replacement might somehow lead to prostate cancer is the big side effect scare in men. It is a situation quite similar to the relationship between estrogen therapy and breast cancer in women, so much so that for much of what follows you might interchange, estrogen, with, testosterone, and, breast, with, prostate.

The FDA Warning

As I quoted earlier, in regard to prostate cancer, the FDA's official position on the use of testosterone is that older men:

"… may be at an increased risk of developing … prostatic carcinoma although conclusive evidence to support this concept is lacking."

It is very important for the patient and the medical practitioner alike to understand the message the FDA is trying to convey here.

"Develop" is not synonymous with "cause". A quick look in the dictionary reveals that develop can indeed mean "to bring into being", but it can also mean "to cause to grow." Fertilizer will stimulate grass to grow, but it will not bring it into being. Testosterone has been on the market for at least fifty-three years, and the only proven relationship between the hormone and prostate cancer is similar to fertilizer and grass.

One final comment on the word the FDA uses to describe the testosterone—prostate cancer relationship, "concept". It is so intriguing because of its ambiguity. There can be a "concept" that anything may cause prostate cancer—perhaps riding a bicycle as a youth—perhaps using a certain brand of condom—perhaps reading or watching too much porn, or not enough. The FDA chooses to put this concept out as a warning to the public, but two other major Federal agencies, the National Cancer Institute and the CDC (Centers for Disease Control and Prevention), don't even mention testosterone in their sections dealing with the possible causes of prostate cancer.

This FDA warning has resulted in the existence of a highly unusual and curious phenomenon surrounding the use of testosterone to treat deficiencies of the hormone. Consider the following:

It is common medical knowledge that testosterone is responsible for muscular strength, energy, and sexuality.

It is also common medical knowledge that ovaries and testes slowly fail as hormone secreting glands as we grow older, and that as a result the level of testosterone in our body declines.

It is common knowledge to everyone that strength, energy and sexuality substantially decline as we grow older.

Surely, if one plus one plus one equals three, the common sense conclusion from these facts, especially in view of the very broad scope of indication the FDA has officially given to men, is that testosterone deficiency is very common and should be routinely treated. If not women, at least millions of men should be getting regular testosterone replacement therapy. They are not. Why not?

One major reason we saw In Chapter Three. The testosterone "normal" laboratory values upon which doctors base their therapeutic judgments are flawed. The other major reason is fear. There is no question but that the vast majority of doctors are afraid to use testosterone. The FDA has put the words "testosterone" and "prostate cancer" together in the same sentence. The fact that "conclusive evidence is lacking" was added to the end of the sentence doesn't make a dent in the apprehension engendered in the medical mind. In our modern world where medical malpractice suits are golden egg laying geese to the legal profession, most doctors don't even want to hear the word "testosterone". That one vague warning sentence, whether an intentional scare tactic, or unintentional, has precluded the medical profession from treating a common, serious, debilitating, disease that is responsible for an unconscionable amount of suffering and death.

The Nature of Prostate Cancer

While I do not believe that testosterone will bring prostate cancer into being, there is no question but that testosterone will accelerate the growth of most prostate cancers. It would, therefore, be expected that any man receiving testosterone who has an as yet undiagnosed prostate cancer will manifest the disease earlier than a similar man not getting testosterone therapy. Studies comparing the incidence of prostate cancer between a group of men getting testosterone treatment and a group of men not getting testosterone, have demonstrated exactly this phenomenon. Initially, the testosterone treated group seems to have a higher incidence of prostate cancer, but what is actually happening is that pre-existing prostate cancers in the testosterone treated group are simply growing a little faster and being diagnosed earlier. As these studies progressed, as more time passed, more and more men in the untreated group began to show their prostate cancers. The incidence numbers gradually evened out until they were essentially identical. In the end there was no higher rate of prostate cancer in the testosterone treated group. They were just getting prostate cancer "fertilizer" for a while.

It isn't likely that prostate cancer victims in this situation have lost anything by having received testosterone treatment. The reader shouldn't necessarily picture such a patient finding himself suddenly riddled with prostate cancer and at death's door. With periodic checking of the PSA, the blood test for prostate cancer, any existing cancer that has been stimulated to grow faster will still be found at an early stage of the disease. In addition, these men have shown that they have the good kind of prostate cancer. When the testosterone is stopped, the commonly used anti-testosterone drugs will obviously be very effective in stopping or markedly slowing the progression of the disease. There is no compelling reason to believe that there would be any significant change in the prognosis of the disease.

My disbelief in the concept that testosterone causes prostate cancer stems from a few sources. Malignant cells are malignant because of their damaged DNA. It doesn't make much sense that a naturally occurring hormone would cause that kind of damage. Most hormones work by attaching to receptors outside the cell, on its membrane, and thereby activate processes inside the cell.

If testosterone did cause prostate cancer the phenomenon of why prostate cancer is exceedingly rare in men who have the highest blood testosterone levels, (ages eighteen to twenty-five), and is seen almost exclusively in older men who have the lowest levels of testosterone, would have to be explained. Indeed, statistics show that the older the man (and the lower the testosterone level), the greater the risk of getting prostate cancer. And where is the higher rate of prostate cancer among all the many professional and amateur athletes and body-builders who've been taking truly massive doses of the hormone for many years?

I do, however, believe that there may well be a causative association between testosterone deficiency and prostate cancer.

What Causes Cancer?

A common thread that seems to bind a lot of cancers together is that they are much more apt to appear on a background of chronic inflammation.

- Smoking predisposes to lung, laryngeal, and throat cancer and certainly causes chronic inflammation of the lungs, larynx, and throat.

- Esophageal cancer is much more common in people who have had years of chronic esophagitis, (heartburn).

- Gastric (stomach) cancer is much more prevalent in people with chronically inflamed stomachs (chronic gastritis).

- Colon cancer is much more common in the presence of chronic colitis.

- Liver cancer is extremely prevalent in the presence of chronic hepatitis and cirrhosis.

- Asbestos in the lung causes chronic inflammation and leads to the cancer called mesothelioma.

- Chronic cervicitis markedly predisposes to cervical cancer.

- Chronic repeated exposure to the sun causes repeated inflammation of the skin and is well known to promote skin cancer.

- It has been reported that there is a higher incidence of gall bladder cancer in people with infected, chronically inflamed, gall bladders.

- Cancer of the bladder is more common in smokers and people who have had frequent exposure to certain chemicals. It is likely that the chemicals in the urine result in a chronic mild bladder inflammation, an entity known as chemical cystitis.

There is a theory that cancer is triggered by damage done to a cell's DNA, its chromosomes, by free radicals. These free radicals are highly chemically reactive compounds continually being formed in the body. There is evidence that they cause ongoing damage to DNA strands, and it is known that mechanisms exist within the cell to repair damaged DNA. It might be that there are a few key spots or types of damage that the cell cannot fix and that alter the DNA in a manner that makes the cell malignant. The damaged cell loses its responsiveness to the mechanisms that regulate cell growth and reproduction, and begins to multiply uncontrollably.

It is known that people can have genes that predispose them to a certain type of cancer. A gene is nothing more than a segment of DNA. The exact sequence of molecules that make up DNA, and, obviously, the segments we call genes, vary from person to person. Having the gene for a certain type of cancer may simply be having a section of DNA that is biochemically more susceptible or vulnerable to being damaged by free radicals. People may also have differing natural abilities to neutralize these free radicals, or to repair their damaged DNA. We see the manifestation of these differences as people having more or less resistance or susceptibility to cancer.

Inflammation is known to markedly increase the production of free radicals, and may likely be the mechanism by which chronic inflammation predisposes to malignancies.

Testosterone Deficiency and Prostate Cancer

How does the above relate to testosterone deficiency and prostate cancer?

As mentioned earlier, just as I've been surprised by the number of younger women who seem to be symptomatic of inadequate testosterone levels, so I believe the same is true with men. There are a lot of men whose active sex life ends at a relatively early age. One of the known consequences of masculine sexual inactivity is prostatitis, prostate infection. Acute prostatitis, for example, is relatively common in men whose wives are suddenly sexually unavailable because of late pregnancy or recent delivery. Mild chronic prostatitis, not severe enough to cause symptoms, is a fairly common phenomenon.

It is not at all unusual to find men with a slightly tender prostate when doing routine rectal examinations.

I propose the possibility of the following sequence of events. A relatively inadequate amount of testosterone in younger men leads to a diminished libido and sexual inactivity at an early age. The retention of prostatic fluid leads to the development of a mild chronic prostatitis. After many years/decades, the chronic prostatic inflammation leads to prostate cancer. This mechanism might also apply to older men. Perhaps even ending sexual activity in the sixties or seventies could cause mild prostatic inflammation and lead to cancer in the seventies or eighties. There might well be a statistical relationship between the end of sexual activity and the onset of prostate cancer.

At the time I wrote the above I thought it was an original supposition. I recently found a prostate cancer website which reported that research done at Case Western Reserve University revealed that chronic prostate inflammation signficantly increased the risk of prostate cancer. This hypothesis makes a lot more sense than the proposition that a natural hormone like testosterone causes cancer when the less of it you have the more common the malignancy.

A thought on the subject of testosterone and men with known prostate cancer.

Almost all men with prostate cancer are treated to essentially eliminate testosterone from their bodies. The concept here is that you don't want to have any fertilizer around living prostate cancer cells. The serious adverse health effects of testosterone deficiency in these men are only first being documented by medical studies. As the population, and these men with prostate cancer, live longer, these hormone deficient health issues are likely going to become more and more consequential.

Any man with a history of prostate cancer may, or may not, have living cancer cells somewhere in his body. They may have all been killed, or they may be dormant for reasons of medical therapy, and be undetectable. If a man with living cancer cells were to receive testosterone therapy, those cells would almost certainly wake up and start to grow. Of course, if such a situation occurred and was detected, the discontinuance of the testosterone and the resumption of anti-testosterone therapy would in all likelihood make the cancer cells dormant again. Possibly, nothing major would have been lost.

It may well be found to be the case that in men with prostate cancer the consequences of profound testosterone deficiency become so devastating as the years pass, that a trial of testosterone therapy becomes less of an ultimate risk to health and life than the continuance of the deficiency state.

9

Menopause, Miscellaneous, and Summary

I'm including a discussion on menopause because it is a very closely related hormone deficient condition as well as the setting for the bulk of testosterone deficiency states in women. In my opinion, as with testosterone deficiency, menopause has not been viewed with intellectual clarity by the medical community. My sentiment can best be described by relating a recent conversation I had with Dr. Gabriel Spergel, an endocrinologist friend of mine. We were chatting in the hospital, discussing some details of my use of testosterone, when he remarked, "I've always consider menopause to be a disease." His statement startled me because it had such a ring of truth to it.

Dr. Spergel went on to say, "Menopause is a disease that should not be permitted to go without treatment. Nature's job is to get rid of us when we are past reproducing, and our job is to maintain vigor, strength, and a good sense of well-being. Menopause is 'natural', but so is plague and cancer."

Menopause is the syndrome caused by the progressive failure of the ovaries to produce quantities of hormones that were normal during an earlier time of life. The consequences of this glandular hormonal failure include loss of the menstrual cycle and reproductive ability, loss of the desire to have sexual relations and the ability to orgasm, an instability in the vascular system that results in episodes of flushing and heat sensations, rapid deterioration of bone tissue, (a process we call osteoporosis), steadily increasing fatigue and muscular weakness, mild to moderate anemia, and very often depression. (*This is not a disease?*) Is it not a disease because every woman goes through it? Every woman, and man also, for that matter, goes through joint degeneration, mental deterioration, vascular blockage, etc., etc., but they are diseases.

Menopause should be regarded as a genetic disease affecting the female of the human species. I think it is an insult to the human female to say to them that all the above is what they must suffer through because it is normal and natural. At the great risk of being excessively repetitive, *almost all diseases are normal and natural.*

The existence of a genetic disease that affects our entire species, every single human being, is not uncommon. Almost all animals make their own ascorbic acid, otherwise known as Vitamin C. Humans cannot, that's why it's a vitamin. We die from scurvy if we don't eat ascorbic acid. Scurvy, therefore, is a genetic disease of mankind. Almost all animals also make their own Vitamin B12. Humans cannot. Again, that's why it's a vitamin. Like scurvy, pernicious anemia (vitamin B12 deficiency) is a genetic disease of the human species.

Needless to say, since I agree with my colleague that menopause is a disease, I have long believed that all women should be taking hormone replacement therapy, both female and male hormones, probably for all or most their lives. Why not try to preserve the basic structure and strength of the body the "natural" way?

Hormonal replacement therapy in women always raises the question of whether estrogen causes breast cancer. I have two positions on the subject. I don't know if it does. I have never believed that it does, and now neither does the National Institute of Health, as will be seen shortly.

When an agent really does incite a malignancy the results of studies on the matter are usually very clear-cut. No serious study ever showed that smoking does not cause lung cancer. No serious study ever showed that asbestos inhalation doesn't cause mesothelioma, or that excessive sun exposure doesn't cause skin cancer. When dealing with estrogens and breast cancer, however, it seems that every other study over the past many decades has come up with opposite findings. There are probably as many studies showing that estrogen does not cause breast cancer as those which supposedly do. The study well publicized a few years ago supposedly suggested a causal relationship, at least at that time, and everyone always assumes that the last study is the valid one, the final word. Of course, every study was the last study in its time.

Like the situation with testosterone and prostate cancer, some things about a cause and effect relationship between estrogen and breast cancer just don't make much sense.

> As with testosterone and prostate cancer, if estrogen causes breast cancer why isn't it more prevalent among younger women who naturally have higher levels of estrogen? Why is it that most breast cancer victims are women at an age when their estrogen levels are declining?

> If estrogen causes breast cancer why aren't we seeing breast cancer in those millions of young women who, for many, many, decades, have been taking estrogen type hormones that are present in oral contraceptives?

Just as with testosterone and prostate cancer, it's obvious that estrogens will make estrogen dependent breast cancers grow faster, and, likewise, anti-estrogen drugs will stop or slow the growth of these tumors. *But just because the hormones promote the growth of a cancer that has still retained some of the biochemical and physiologic characteristics of its parent tissue doesn't mean that the hormone can actually trigger the malignancy into being.*

I can postulate a cause of breast cancer related to the inflammation theory. Past studies have shown that women who breast-feed have a lower rate of breast cancer than women who do not breast-feed. The differences have not been very dramatic. I wonder if those types of studies have been carried far enough. Has anyone compared the rate of breast cancer to the number of weeks of breast-feeding during a reproductive lifetime? Women who birth a child or two and breast feed for a few months might have quite different statistics than women who have six or seven children and breast feed each for a year or more.

It is the case with breasts as with prostate glands, the more frequently and consistently they are emptied, the healthier they are.

Subsequent to writing the above I decided to look at the actual numbers reported in the recent study that has kept millions of women from taking hormone replacement therapy. I was so astounded I had to double check the findings at the National Institute of Health web site.

What Exactly Did That Estrogen Study Show?

The study that was in the news a few years ago that indicted estrogen as a cause of breast cancer and heart disease was the Women's Health Initiative. It stopped millions of post-menopausal women from taking estrogen, and is the prime reason women are not taking estrogen replacement therapy today. The following is the essence of that study taken from an FDA approved blurb which is included in products containing estrogen and is easily available online.

The study was a comparison of women taking estrogen or an estrogen—progesterone combination, to women taking a placebo (a pill containing no active medication). These are the reported results of the total study.

	@ 8,000 women given a <u>placebo</u>	@ 8,000 women given <u>estrogen</u>
Heart disease problems	30	37
Strokes	30	38
Breast Cancer	30	38
Colon cancer	16	10
Uterus cancer	6	5
Death from other causes	40	37
Total death rate	No difference	

Out of sixteen thousand women there were seven more cases of heart trouble and eight more cases of breast cancer among the eight thousand that were taking estrogen. I personally don't see that as proof of anything. There were also six *less* cases of colon cancer among the women taking estrogen. All in all there was one (1) more case of cancer in the eight thousand estrogen treated women, and absolutely no difference in the death rate. In other words, you'll live just as long whether you take estrogen or not. These are the numbers that have made millions of women elect to suffer the uncomfortable, depressing, debilitating, and sometimes devastating, effects of menopause. But that's not the end of the story.

There was another part of that same study that wasn't advertised as well. It was a sub-study which compared women taking estrogen alone to women taking a placebo. These are the reported heart disease and breast cancer results of the sub-study.

	@ 5,000 women given a <u>placebo</u>	@ 5,000 women given <u>estrogen</u>
Heart disease problems	56	53
Breast Cancer	34	28

The National Institute of Health has judged that the *lower* incidence of heart disease and the *lower* incidence of breast cancer among women <u>taking</u> estrogen is not significant. Their conclusion:

"Estrogen-alone hormone therapy does not increase the risk of breast cancer in postmenopausal women, according to an updated analysis of the breast cancer findings of the Women's Health Initiative (WHI) Estrogen-Alone Trial."

We have a situation now where the overwhelming majority of doctors, in New York at least, are advising their female patients to not take estrogen supplements because of the possibility of breast cancer, while the N.I.H. has stated that estrogen has been proven to *not* cause breast cancer.

It would seem that those responsible for the W.H.I. study had a hair-trigger impulse to terminate it at even the slightest hint of a possibility of some adverse outcome.

There is one more aspect of menopausal hormone replacement to be mentioned. If women only take female hormones for menopausal therapy it is possible that they could experience a further reduction in the secretion of ovarian male hormones. The pituitary gland senses the increased estrogen level coming from the pills and decreases its stimulation of ovarian hormone secretion. This situation commonly leads to women being free of excessive flushing and excessive vaginal dryness, but having no sexual desire at all and an inability to have orgasms.

MISCELLANEOUS

I have a couple of observations and a conjecture to relate here.

It seems that maybe testosterone therapy can cause the elderly to regain their taste for meat and other protein foods. The description of an elderly diet as being, "tea and toast", goes back to my medical school days. Older people do lose their taste for high protein foods. Protein is the construction material of the body. As I've stated before, nature does common sense things, even if we don't always see the sense behind it at first.

Without sufficient testosterone our bodies are "catabolic", they are deteriorating, disintegrating. Bones are thinning, muscles are shrinking and weakening, red blood cell levels are falling, etc., etc. If the body isn't building anything it doesn't need much protein. A homebuilder isn't going to buy lumber if the carpenters have stopped working.

When we replace the missing testosterone "anabolism", construction, begins again. Bones and muscles begin to rebuild, red blood cell production increases. It's as if the carpenters suddenly reappeared and began yelling at the builder, "We need plywood! We need studs and plasterboard!" If our bodies go into a rebuilding mode we are going to need supplies of protein, and nature apparently re-awakens that taste. The loss of the taste for protein in the older population may be yet another manifestation of the disease of testosterone deficiency.

The second observation is that testosterone deficiency may result in a degree of cold intolerance. Some patients, prior to starting therapy, have told me that they never used to feel this cold. One person on therapy experienced a degree of heat intolerance, almost always feeling warmer than others around him. Of course, thyroid hormone deficiency is well known to result in cold intolerance, and that is certainly a disease.

My conjecture concerns my reference, early in the book, to the deleterious consequences of high doses of cortisone. It does seem that many of the effects of cortisone and testosterone are opposing, such as on osteoporosis and muscle strength, and, I believe, type II diabetes. High doses of cortisone are sometimes necessary in a number of diseases. The therapy is often unavoidable. I wonder if any study has been done to determine if the simultaneous administration of effective doses of testosterone with cortisone does anything to ameliorate the negative side effects of the cortisone.

SUMMARY

Medicine has made enormous strides since I became part of it some forty-five years ago. The modern treatments to prevent one of the two most common causes of death, namely vascular disease in the form of heart attacks and strokes, are highly safe and effective. These drugs to control blood pressure, cholesterol, and diabetes will be adding years, maybe even decades, to the lives of those wise enough to take advantage of them. Great gains are also being made on the other major cause of death, cancer. Strategies to prevent, diagnosis early and cure, and drugs to keep as yet incurable cancer under control, are becoming more and more effective every year. But while we can look forward to a longer life span, how will we feel during those added years? If we do not address the issue of those hormone deficiencies coming from failed ovaries and testes, our added time on this Earth is not going to be as rewarding or fruitful as it might be.

If we are going to take the best possible care of ourselves we also have to get rid of the notions that normal and natural are always desirable states. They have to be examined critically, as does the nonsensical concept that if we only ate right, exercised, and took herbs, we would all enjoy perpetual good health.

When it comes to testosterone, or rather the lack of, I see a disease that can significantly affect younger people sexually and socially, as well as possibly predispose to prostate cancer. It may also be a cause of the Chronic Fatigue Syndrome.

In the older segment of the population the deficiency eats away women's bones, and causes significant anemia, muscle weakness, fatigue, and depression. I believe that the combination of these factors can cause or worsen congestive heart failure, and increases the aged predisposition to develop pneumonia and other respiratory problems. I believe it is *a* prime cause of the general deterioration of the aged. The simple replacement of this hormone can have multiple beneficial effects and result in profound improvement in the quality and quantity of life.

We need a thorough re-evaluation of the consequences of testosterone deficiency.

We need to revise the blood level ranges that we consider to be "normal" so they reflect reality and do not hide deficiency states.

We need to recognize the sexuality of human beings, the physical, emotional, and social importance of it, and the primary role played by testosterone.

About the Author

Dr. Barry Gordon received his M.D. degree from the Chicago Medical School in 1965. He completed his training in Internal Medicine at the Jewish Hospital and Medical Center in Brooklyn in 1968, and in Hematology at the Montefiore Hospital Medical Center in the Bronx in 1969. Dr. Gordon has served as Chief of Hematology at two Brooklyn hospitals, and has been on the teaching staff of the Downstate Medical School (SUNY Health and Science Center at Brooklyn) as a Clinical Instructor in Medicine. Most of Dr. Gordon's career has been devoted to his Internal Medicine/Primary Care practice in Brooklyn which he continues to maintain. He is the author of, *Get Well, Stay Well.*

978-0-595-41494-9
0-595-41494-X

25519071R00097

Made in the USA
Lexington, KY
26 August 2013